Advance Praise for
The Pro-Aging Playbook

"I could write a novel about Dr. Paul Jarrod Frank's dermatological knowledge and expertise on how to get your skin looking its best. But his main attraction for me is what he knows and says all the time: You are only as beautiful as you feel on the inside! Dr. Frank reminds us that while he can help us to a point, we have to remember what's most important and do the deeper work as well."

—MADONNA

"A few shots here and there may help on the surface, but Dr. Paul Jarrod Frank taught us that wellness and beauty must start from within for it to truly reflect on the outside. A completely new approach to aging, *The Pro-Aging Playbook* offers a wealth of insight, tools, and tips on how to look and feel your very best."

—MARC JACOBS & CHAR DEFRANCESCO

"I have had the extraordinary opportunity of watching Dr. Paul Jarrod Frank grow within the skincare and beauty industry. Success for him was not an overnight achievement, but a journey in truly mastering his holistic approach to beauty, skin, and overall lifestyle. He believes in treating the whole body to obtain the results you want for your skin and external beauty, and not just going straight into cosmetic procedures. To feel good on the outside you must feel good on the inside. He practices what he preaches by eating healthy, not drinking during the week, meditating, and exercising. I understand why so many turn to him for insight and advice. What he teaches truly resonates with so many people! I am beyond lucky to call him a friend."

—RACHEL ZOE

"Dr. Paul Jarrod Frank has devoted his life and career to helping people feel beautiful inside and out. In his new book, he teaches us that true beauty is an inside job. I love how he combines personal growth methods with the latest dermatological options to help readers look and feel their best."

—GABRIELLE BERNSTEIN, #1 *New York Times* bestselling author

"Dr. Paul Jarrod Frank is so much more than a dermatologist. He's someone who has the power to help you manifest your best self—body and mind—so that you glow from within. This book is the start of your journey."

—JESSICA MATLIN, Beauty Director, *Harper's BAZAAR*

"Feeling good and looking good go hand in hand. It's important to share your best self with the world, and I've relied on top beauty experts, including Dr. Paul Jarrod Frank, to keep me looking my best just as others have relied on me. This holistic, educational look at beauty and wellness from a top industry expert is a must-read."

—SALLY HERSHBERGER, Hair Legend

"We all know the saying 'beauty starts on the inside,' but aging certainly does, as well. Dr. Paul Jarrod Frank has given us a roadmap to become our best selves by taking a more holistic approach and looking at the whole picture—from calming our minds with meditation to examining what, when, and even why we eat. I found this book to be not only informative, but also very inspirational. A must-read for anyone who wants to feel and look their best (and who doesn't want that?)."

—KATIE LEE, Bestselling Cookbook Author & Television Food Critic

THE
PRO-AGING
PLAYBOOK

THE PRO-AGING PLAYBOOK

EMBRACING A LIFESTYLE OF BEAUTY AND WELLNESS INSIDE AND OUT

PAUL JARROD FRANK, MD

Post Hill
PRESS

Post Hill Press
New York • Nashville
posthillpress.com

Published in the United States of America

For Ann, my sister and unsung hero

Contents

Preface

Beauty always shines from within. It is human to want
to give it the reflection it deserves.

—DR. PAUL JARROD FRANK

I've got some good news and some bad news.

The bad news first: no matter how hard you work out, how much
you eat right, or how well you take care of yourself, we're all going
to the same place.

Now the good news: everybody's aging—it's epidemic—and
it's certainly better than the alternative. If you're breathing, you're
achieving! Not only that, but we're living in an era where we can
influence how we age, physically and mentally, which is kind of
astonishing when you think about it. Modern science, vaccines,
indoor plumbing, antibiotics, and good nutrition, among many
other modern innovations, have given us the luxury of being able
to live long enough to see the wrinkles form on our faces and feel
the progressive and natural decrease in functioning of our bodies
and senses.

But is living longer enough? What about living *better*?

Just because we're getting older doesn't mean we can't be
vital, feel beautiful, and remain positive about the future. Youth,
as the saying goes, is wasted on the young. Being young is easy;

you don't get credit for it. Getting older is a gift, and it's up to you to make the best of it.

This was exemplified by one of my favorite patients, who started coming to me every three months when she was *ninety*. Yes, *ninety*! She wore big glasses and needed a walker, but other than that, you'd have thought she was in her late sixties. She was sharp as a tack, and after every appointment she'd say, "If you don't see me in three months, Doc, you know where I'll be." All she wanted me to do was put some filler in her cheeks to lift her face and jawline a bit—it made her happy. "People are always asking me why I come to you and do this and do that, and I tell them it's better than going to any other doctor," she said to me one day, when she was ninety-four. "Most of my friends go to doctors all day and then they're in the graveyard. I don't want people treating me like I'm ninety-four—I don't *feel* ninety-four. I might move slow and old, but I don't *think* slow and old. What you do makes me feel good, and when I feel good, people treat me different. I want to look seventy, not ninety-four, you know?"

She would always smile widely, and her demeanor made me happy and gave me guidance and perspective. I knew, each time I saw her, that the best form of cosmetic surgery is a *smile*—and that is something you can't necessarily inject.

A lot of people don't look as good as they feel inside. This patient still *felt* young. I didn't make her look decades younger. I made her feel more *vital*. That was exactly what she wanted; it served her sense of self. She is the epitome of pro-aging. Feeling better about herself in the mirror made her more functional—not just for herself, but for everybody in her orbit. The way we treat ourselves affects how other people treat us too.

On the other hand, I had a new patient who was only fifty, yet she repeatedly told me how *old* she felt. She, by no means, looked it. "You know the best part about you?" I asked, because it was clear her issues were more emotional than physical. She shook her head. "The one thing that's never going to age is your eye color. You have gorgeous green eyes, and all I have to do is put a frame around them. That's the easy part. The hard part is seeing all that you have already."

I wasn't focusing her attention on the hollowing of her cheeks or some lines on her forehead. That's *my* job. I wanted to enhance her good parts and for her to take stock of what she already possessed. In the end, she was thrilled, because it's my job to make people feel good about what I can do for them instead of making them feel like they're *old* and need to be fixed.

In other words, pro-aging is the opposite of anti-aging: It's a change of perspective.

With a pro-aging attitude, you can't just do one thing—go work out *or* go to a cosmetic dermatologist *or* go to a psychologist *or* go to a nutritionist. You have to do a little bit of everything. Someone who eats well and gets enough sleep, for example, will metabolize their calories differently than someone who eats the exact same meals but barely sleeps due to stress. Or someone who eats well and regularly meditates but does no exercise will find it hard to be strong and fit.

A lot of my patients tell me, "Ohmigod, I want to do treatments that will make me look like you." I'm fifty, but they think I look years younger *only* because I can treat myself with the very best that cosmetic technology has to offer. But, in truth, my patients aren't responding just to my skin, but to my *mood*—my vigor and my vitality.

From 8:00 a.m. to 6:00 p.m. I'm on a stage, performing for my patients because I want them to absorb my energy. When I'm not feeling my best, didn't get a good night's sleep, or was unfocused during my daily meditation, I know that will not only affect my personality, but even what I'm giving my patients via the needle or laser.

So how do I keep my energy up? I try to live my life like a professional athlete. I don't drink during the week. I exercise nearly every day. I meditate twice a day. I watch what I eat. I'm realistic about what I need and want.

Part of my success is not just how good I am at what I do, but my life balance. How I live is attainable to anybody, but I am not an unwavering monk and I go off-balance at times too. The stereotype of the most successful person used to be someone who doesn't have to sleep, doesn't have to eat, and works nonstop. Someone telling me they only need four hours of sleep is not impressive. Instead, it tells me that person is scatterbrained, multitasking, and unhealthy, with a shortened lifespan.

In fact, the most successful people I know want to share how they meditate, how well they sleep, and how well they eat. They don't just take the time to achieve professionally, they take the time to pro-age *holistically*. They know that success and pro-aging have nothing to do with money—it's all about how to get the harmonious balance by creating new habits to look better, feel better, and live longer.

You'll see how to find that balance in this book. You won't feel deprived or hungry or angry at yourself if you miss a workout or eat too much on vacation. I never use the word *cheat*. Instead, you *treat*! We deserve to spoil ourselves sometimes.

People tend to think that if they exercise all the time and starve themselves and wear designer clothes, they're going to be skinny and perfect and desirable, and that if I treat them with the newest device, or if they put the trendiest cream on their face, they're going to be beautiful. My answer is different: What they need is sleep, exercise, reset time, and to kick-start their eating habits, or they're wasting their time with me. They don't realize it's much more to do with what's between their ears than anything else! And that the visual feedback we get from looking at people or at ourselves has a direct connection to what's going on inside the body. Doing what you can to look your best will absolutely affect you internally. That's what pro-aging is all about.

I firmly believe that both the inside as well as our visible façade are intricately connected and influence one another on every possible level. My expertise and guidance as an "exterior designer" is, by no means, the most essential to the many assets of the pro-aging lifestyle you'll learn about. My work is merely an important piece of this wonderful puzzle.

I do believe that anyone and everyone can benefit from any level of the cosmetic options available to make them feel better about themselves. As an expert in the beauty field, I'm writing this book to tell you that "beauty" is a very important component of the wellness industry, of everyone's well-being, and that it has been left out of the conversation. Despite the fact that we don't want to over-focus on how we look, how we appear to ourselves and others is an integral part of every other aspect of life. It's the elephant in the room that most people in the wellness industry and the rest of the world are not willing to acknowledge.

During my training, I had a professor who was a renowned expert in hair transplant surgery, and he dedicated a lot of his time to teaching about hair loss and how to effectively treat it medically and surgically. Funnily enough, he was very bald and was often asked why he didn't do any hair restorative treatments on himself. His answer was always the same: "There are two types of balding patients," he'd explain. "People who suffer from baldness and those that are just bald. I am just bald."

This amplifies my point that how we perceive ourselves in the mirror differs for everyone. For most, the reflection does have some impact on how we feel, but how *much* of it influences us is the big variable. Hair, noses, wrinkles, birthmarks, or toes—we all see ourselves through our own worthy lenses.

I often have patients come in and, when asked what I can do for them, respond with, "Dr. Frank, what do I *need* to do?"

I tell them: "What you *need* to do is to go home and look in the mirror and feel positive about who you are. What you *need* to do is find happiness on the inside, take stock of the assets you have, and be grateful." Then I pause, smile, and add, "Once you've done that, then I've got a lot of tricks for you to make your outside reflect your inside."

The point here is that there are no Botox shots or lasers that will take away people's unhappiness or insecurities. I'm merely a piece of a puzzle. It's a very important piece, and it's amazing that the technology exists to give people quick fixes. But I'm the icing on the cake—which is always the best part of the cake, in my opinion.

Now, I know what you're thinking: This celebrity cosmetic dermatologist is going to start talking about and selling all the supposed quick fixes of injections, lasers, and surgery that will wipe away all the insecurities of aging. I wish it were that easy, but it's not. Does this mean it's hard? No, it does not.

You just have to be *pro* about it.

Anti-aging is merely a sales term used by companies to scare you into buying their products. Anti-aging is also a kickback to the negative connotation, burned into the psychology, marketing, and publicity of the society we live in, that aging is a bad thing. That you need to *fix* it. That you need to purchase, market, inject, cut, detoxify, and do anything you can to stop it.

This is how my colleagues and I were trained, but I soon realized that an enormous rejection led me to upend that training into my pro-aging philosophy.

When the time came to make plans for my future, my parents made their expectations clear that I should go to medical school. My dad was a dentist and my mom was a nurse, and I was almost a little rebellious about their stance until I realized the decision was my own. My parents had always been completely supportive of my academic growth, and I realized that their push for me to go into medicine was not selfish, but something they felt was best for my personality and skills, because they lived it. For them, the field of medicine was one where you could go to sleep at night doing well for yourself and knowing you're also doing well for other people. The health profession provided my parents with a sense of contribution, accomplishment, and lifestyle that suited them well. I was given enormous opportunities, with a supportive family and a private-school education, but as a student, I rarely fulfilled my potential in those formative years. My grades were average, and I only managed to squeak by at the end. I usually appeared distracted, which prevented me from reaching my full aptitude. Nowadays, this would most likely be called attention deficit disorder, but regardless of the cause, I was simply not focused when I needed to be. As a result, when I applied to many different medical schools, I didn't get into any of them. Not one.

I was devastated because, for the first time, I was stricken with the sense of true failure.

When I sat down with myself and admitted that my road to success was going to be paved with hard work and not inheritance, those rejections became the jolt I needed. In retrospect, this led to a spectacular turning point in my life, a deeply ingrained setback that I would never trade for anything. I spent the next year doing postgraduate studies at Columbia University, and from then on, I was top of my class. I got into one medical school, New York Medical College, off the wait list. When I was applying to choose my residency, I was told I was wasting my energy and talents by going into such a highly competitive field as dermatology—one that wasn't of much "significance"—but I ignored the comments. I was an aesthetic, creative person and was already interested in the nascent technologies of skin care.

My mother actually put the dermatology seed in my head. She always knew people prioritized skin problems more than other health issues. As a hospital nurse and an Italian mother, she would indulge me with stories of how dermatologists weren't often called to the hospital, but when they were, they appeared to be the best-dressed and most rested. That seemed good enough for her son. I had studied psychology throughout college and at the time had inklings that I would pursue it professionally.

When I discovered dermatology, what was most curious to me wasn't just the beauty and health of skin, but the psychology of the skin we live in. And, surprisingly, dermatology was merely glanced over in medical-school curriculum. Most physicians knew very little about the largest and most visible organ of the human body. How could that be? People go to the dermatologist more quickly for a spot on their skin than to a cardiologist for a pain in their chest. I knew it was my calling.

My drive and expertise in the subspecialty of cosmetic dermatology developed rapidly. I was given opportunities with great mentors, great training, and enormous support from those close to me. But, despite my early success, it was still frustrating as the field was perceived and sold as a niche specialty preying only on the vain and insecure. It had not yet hit the mainstream, but, even back then, I knew that what I do isn't just about looks. It's about *health* and *lifestyle* and *self-perception*—all key components to the overall quality of our existence.

That's when pro-aging became my life.

We all want guidance. The reason why any industry is filled with guides to this, that, and the other is because that's what people clamor for. When my wife was pregnant with our first baby, we had books stacked up to the ceiling about raising infants, toddlers, and children. My mom—who was an obstetrical nurse—came over one day and tried not to laugh. "Paul," she said, "if there was only one way to take care of a baby, there would only be one book."

There are so many different beauty tips and diets and perspectives and cosmetic applications and books and websites and tweets and postings from pros and amateurs, experts and quacks, and every one of them is there to tout their own kind of guidance.

I want to protect you from all that chatter. I'm not here to tell you what the best answers are to all your beauty and wellness questions, but I'm going to give you my medically sound knowledge, and the most successful options, so you can make pro-aging a part of your life.

Beauty is accessible to everybody, and this book gives you a system that works at home. It might not be as potent as what you'd get from a dermatologist, but I'll bet that every aspect of pro-aging is going to be better than what you're doing now! Modern medicine has taught us how to stay alive at any cost. We've spent too much money on keeping everyone alive and not enough time and energy on improving the quality of that time.

This book is about empowerment. People complain about aging all the time, but we have the opportunity to feel, look, and love better at any age by focusing on the quality, not the quantity of life. This is *not* what you're told or sold in the beauty and wellness industries. Instead, these industries are mired in enormous amounts of marketing and content that are not necessarily effective and can actually be harmful. And there's an enormous amount of quackery.

After two decades as a cosmetic dermatologist, I'm using my expertise as a physician navigating the same challenges as all healthy adults to show you how to be the best version of yourself. I'm not just talking the talk, I'm walking the walk. If you follow me on social media (@drpauljarrodfrank), I'm constantly putting up posts that have nothing to do with cosmetic surgery...simply because I feel like it's my responsibility to help all consumers have a medically informed filter and guide. In the health and wellness community, there are so many wonderful, valuable things to do that will help you sleep, eat, exercise, meditate, and feel better. When I mention nutrition, sleeping habits, and meditation to my patients, they're often shocked at first. But then they realize that pro-aging isn't just about having me do something *to* them. It's about them doing what they need to for themselves as well.

I spend so much time talking to my patients about what works and what doesn't that they've often asked me to write a book with more detailed information. I want you to use this book as a virtual consultation—an at-home version of my expertise.

It doesn't have to be confusing. So here it is!

The Pro-Aging Philosophy

Pro-aging is harnessing the power of all the components of your existence—the way you look, the way you feel, your health and well-being, your sense of self, your relationships, the control of your ego—so you can be the best version of yourself. Once you become an active participant in your own pro-aging, you'll quickly see that it's *proven* and *pro*tective. The results are *pro*found.

Aging isn't just about the loss of looks and functioning. It's also about developing experience, wisdom, perspective, and confidence that only the prescriptions of time can provide. So it ain't all bad!

Still, we live in a world where we're made to feel bad about ourselves as we get older, and the only way to feel better is when someone—who's going to charge us—can fix it. I'm in that world... except my philosophy is not derogatory by telling you what's wrong with you. I'm trying to enhance and make the best of what you've already got. If you don't believe in what you already have, all the enhancement in the world isn't going to make you feel good about yourself. The less you do is sometimes the more you do. Don't always add—sometimes subtract! I'm the last person who'll overdo or oversell. There is always a lot I can do, but it has to come from the right place: from you. Subtle change is significant. Which is why my goal is to show you how to live better longer, not necessarily make you look younger.

Pro-aging is harnessing the power of all components of your existence—the way you look, the way you feel, your health and well-being, your sense of self, your relationships, the control of your ego—so you can be the best version of yourself.

Getting older is a journey that takes effort and deserves credit for work well done. So what do we do about improving the quality of our time while we're alive, as well as our perception, our relationships with people and with our careers, and our self-worth?

Pro-aging is not *anti*-aging.

Pro Is the First Part of *Proactive*

Being proactive by taking the best possible care of yourself is the most powerful thing you can do for your health. There's no overnight miracle to do this. It's the first rule of medicine (and should be the first rule of life).

Part of being your best self is living in a good, healthy body. Our bodies are smarter than we think. In every aspect of pro-aging, the basic premise is to let your body do its job. Everything in beauty and science and medicine is not about what you do, but how you do it.

Living better is not only feeling good—it's also looking good. Our brains weren't genetically programmed to look at ourselves as old and healthy. Hundreds of years ago, when you looked sick, you felt sick. When you were healthy, you looked vital and vibrant. These are not independent concepts. Many people get sexier as they get older—it's the way they carry themselves with confidence, and how they smile. There's nothing worse than a patient who's young, gorgeous, and insecure.

I was a pudgy kid with bad habits and didn't get fit and trim until I was a teenager. Many of my patients never felt beautiful when they were younger and actually start to feel their most attractive as they get older. This is a perception thing. You can be beautiful, and it has nothing to do with comparing yourself to a professional athlete or a Victoria's Secret model. It's about finding some way—the pro-aging way—to get to your best version of yourself.

Pro Is the First Part of *Productive*

With most healthy adults, we now have the amazing capacity to dramatically influence the nature of our aging—not just in how we look, but in how we feel and function. It's astonishing what we can produce when we change our mindset. Every day, my patients tell me that getting old is a bitch. My reflexive comment is always, "Aren't we so lucky to live in an age with such amazing medical advancements? We have technologies and insights for everything from nutrition and fitness to lasers and injectable treatments. A few hundred years ago, we would be lucky to be alive past thirty, let alone have intact white teeth, clear skin, and clean hair. And the toothpaste, organic cleanser, and shampoo to help keep them that way."

Pro Is the First Part of *Progress*

It might sound contrarian, but there are plenty of times when you should actually stop *adding* to your beauty and health regimen, and *subtract* instead.

Less is often more, and small changes are often the way to go. The way to progress is with baby steps. Because they all add up, and because bingeing or starving doesn't work, whether with exercise, with food, with alcohol, with Botox. I do a little bit of exercise almost every day. That's more than enough. I'm not looking to become a professional trainer or a body builder, or to become a robotic version of my younger self.

Making small changes is actually an enormous shift from the way dermatologists and plastic surgeons used to treat their patients. Thirty years ago, you waited until you were of a certain age, and then you'd have an aggressive chemical peel or facelift, need to hide from the world for two or three weeks as you suffered through a painful recuperation, and, hopefully, be good for ten years or so. Now, technological advances have transformed this kind of drastic, risk-filled treatment. My patients always ask, for whatever treatment they want, how long it's going to last. That's the wrong question. Instead, they should ask, "How often do you need to see me to keep me looking my very best?" For most of my patients in their twenties and thirties, I'll see them twice a year on average. In their forties, two or three times a year. In their fifties, three to four times a year; over that, maybe four to six times a year. This doesn't mean that they come in for a total overhaul every time. Instead, it's *maintenance*. I want people to metaphorically color their roots frequently, rather than grow out and reprocess their hair from scratch.

You can't work out, eat right, get in shape, lose weight, and then expect your transformation to magically sustain itself. Maybe you're not training as hard as you did to lose twenty pounds, but you've got to keep doing it. There are no diets that work; there are no exercise routines that you can just do for two months; and there's no form of grooming or cosmetic rejuvenation that you can do and never have to do it again. Even the most aggressive facelift wears off after a decade or so.

This is why you can't be a perfectionist. New patients sit down and announce that they want to get rid of things—bags under their eyes or wrinkles on their cheeks. And my answer is *absolutely not*. This is rarely what they expect to hear! But I add that my goal is to make whatever is bothering them significantly better. We don't want to push the limits. I don't want to do anything that's going to make them look fake or done. I do say no a *lot*, because I don't want to do treatments that won't work well, because everything costs time and money, and everything carries some degree of risk.

> *You need to feel comfortable with the reality of maintenance— you've got to get the idea out of your head that there is a finish line to anything in life.*

You need to feel comfortable with the reality of maintenance— you've got to get the idea out of your head that there is a finish line to anything in life.

Pro-aging isn't just about moisturizing your skin or getting rid of wrinkles. It's having a holistic view of your body and how to take care of yourself. Most of all, the profound changes you're going to see and feel aren't about erasing the years—they're about regaining and optimizing your *vitality*. My patients who hit fifty and feel like they look their best have outgrown the need for comparisons. It has nothing to do with the mirror; it has to do with confidence in themselves. You'll never feel beautiful unless you develop your own inner mirror.

This type of self-actualization is something recognized and exemplified by Madonna, with whom I had the good fortune of spending time with while working on her skincare line, MDNA Skin. She lives life literally and figuratively in forward kinetic motion. What she has accomplished in music, fashion, film, and life is about manifesting her chosen vision and empowering her self-worth. She takes risks and moves forward without second-guessing in self-judgment, despite decades of outside criticism. No great accomplishment is without risk. That's how she looks at beauty, as well. There is no kowtowing to a stereotype of trying to satisfy others, thinking that's possible only by trying to look younger. It's about making herself feel strong and beautiful, leading by example. She epitomizes pro-aging.

Pro-aging is about simplification and filtration of all the content bombarding you, and part of that is telling you what's garbage science and what's not. You don't need genetic testing to figure out which workout is going to be better for you; you don't need designer vitamins; and you don't need to spend a fortune on thirty different moisturizers that won't erase your age spots but will lighten your wallet.

There's no wrong way of making good choices. Every good choice you make is better than nothing, and every small step you take contributes to the bigger picture of looking and feeling your best. This is true whether you're seeing a dermatologist, choosing a new serum, or taking a long walk for your health. You'd be shocked at how a lot of small changes will make very big differences.

Forget extremes. Pro-aging is about new ways to harness the good and minimize the bad.

Pro-Aging Is Not Independent of Wellness

Discussing that provocative word "vanity" with my friends and patients often leads to automatic and erroneous assumptions... just as the word "beauty" leads to the assumption that it's only about a particular kind of physical attractiveness.

What's wonderful about the changing face of cosmetic dermatology is that there's no one beauty standard anymore. People come in all shapes, colors, and sizes, and there's beauty to be found in all of them. We're seeing so many different shades of people, and I don't mean just in terms of color. I mean in terms of sexual orientation, gender identification, comfort in different clothes, makeup, and hairstyles. We still have a long way to go to becoming a full open-minded society, but at least we're not living in the 1950s, when everyone seemingly had the same haircut and lived in segregated communities.

For me, though, beauty isn't so much visual as it is a *feeling*, inside and out, of the way we want to live. It's not based on external standards; it's more of a neurochemical sensation.

Beauty is also a sense of well-being, of feeling good about yourself. It's not necessarily related to other people's judgment. That's one of the hardest things for people to separate from, because they see their beauty only in terms of how other people respond to it—but it's really the internalization or the emotional effect that is most important here.

I have patients that are not empirically beautiful people, but what I do for them makes them feel very good about themselves. I also have patients who are drop-dead gorgeous and who make a living from their looks. Sadly, no matter what I do, many of them continue to feel ugly. They don't need more Botox—but they may well need some self-reassessment. And I try to help them, as I help all my patients, define *their* version of beauty.

Another vitally important aspect of pro-aging I discuss is about directing your energy into *feeling* beautiful, which is a positive thought.

We spend so much of our lives being caught up in negative thinking. Mostly because we are being often sold solutions to negatives: why this car is better than what you have, or why this product will detoxify you, or how that cosmetic procedure will make you look less old. Whether you're treating yourself to a new car or a syringe full of filler, the potential of fulfillment in that choice has to do, as with all things, with the attitude you take going into it. Realization and appreciation for what you already have may make these choices more fulfilling as an added bonus to your life or well-being.

Point being, part of being and feeling beautiful and being the best version of yourself is about perspective and training yourself in removing negative thought patterns. Not just negative thought patterns about yourself—*all* negative thought patterns, as we live in a world filled with discontent. Discontent with politics, discontent with media, discontent with what we see online, discontent with ourselves, our jobs, our bodies, our peers...you get the point. People are constantly choosing to channel unhappiness about things. Now I am certainly not saying we should just choose to smile and accept the inequalities of the world and not strive for resolutions and improvements in ourselves and our surroundings—but the way we choose to do it can be so much more effective by *how* we do it. Time spent bashing politicians on Twitter may not be as productive as time spent being supportive of those politicians we admire. If people in your life are annoying, don't waste your time gossiping about them; address the conflict directly or just put your energy into relationships you want to build instead.

And if you want to make self-improvement of yourself physically through cosmetic procedures, you can't come from a place thinking that you are old or unattractive and a few needles will magically undo that feeling. They won't.

Self-Love Is Not Vanity—It's What Makes Us Beautiful

Too often, we spend too much time beating ourselves up in this world. About our looks, about how we spend our time, about our bad habits, about the choices we wish we hadn't made. That's just human nature. The world is a very challenging place—which is why self-love is the most necessary step to feeling beautiful. Because if you don't love yourself, you can't love how you look.

Especially when it comes to discussing the concept of *vanity*.

Everyone talks about wellness, but not about *beauty* as an integral part of it. This is an issue I discuss with my patients every day. The beauty and wellness industry is hamstrung by its misguided notion of vanity. The perception years ago, which was true, was that you were especially vain if you wanted cosmetic surgery. Sometimes, back then, whatever limited cosmetic surgeries existed were expensive; they were more dangerous; they necessitated a lot of downtime; the results could be freaky. So, understandably, it was not very wise to put yourself at risk and deplete your bank account just for vanity.

Pro-aging wants you to upend your notion of vanity. Make it a positive as opposed to a negative by focusing your self-care on the inside *and out*. The pro-aging lifestyle is realizing that function and aesthetics are intrinsically dependent on each other. Everything that helps you functionally helps you look better, and everything that helps you look better helps you functionally.

> *Everything that helps you functionally helps you look better, and everything that helps you look better helps you functionally.*

In other words, people think that the way you look only has to do with the way you take care of your skin, the style of your hair, and so on. They generally don't realize that food, exercise, and meditation have equal influence. My job is to help people integrate beauty into their lives both aesthetically and functionally—this is what always get the best results.

How to do that? By first realizing that not always feeling good about the way you look or caring about how you look is not a psychological disease. It's not narcissism. It's *not* vanity. It's not about believing you're more or less beautiful or better than anybody else. It's about recognizing who you are and who you want to be.

John Demsey, executive group president of the Estée Lauder Companies, a close friend and old boss from my early brand-ambassador days, would always say, "Beauty is a universal aspiration. Everyone in the world wants to look their best, feel their best, and project themselves forward. No one thinks they look too good. No one thinks they couldn't take a little advice or do a bit better. This constant striving for fulfillment, or this aspiration for perfection or putting one's best self forward, regardless of your orientation, goes back to the beginning of humanity."

I've mentioned already that we weren't meant to live as long as many people do now. Science keeps us alive and feeling relatively well, and we want the mirror, the reflection, to match that. So I want you to think of vanity as a reward for the hard work you put into your self-care. Because beauty is always in the eyes of the beholder, and the most important set of eyes will always be your own.

Nor should aesthetic rejuvenation be considered vanity. Cosmetic procedures are now no different than grooming. In the 1930s, you'd get your hair colored in the basement of the salon because there was such a stigma about it. Who doesn't color or bleach their hair now? And, of course, you shave your armpits or paint your nails. You get your teeth whitened or veneers put on. You don't think about it; it's just part of your daily routine.

I don't really look at Botox, fillers, lasers as anything else other than an extension of all of these things we do every day to groom or beautify ourselves. Millennials are the first generation who consider rejuvenation as a form of grooming, like going for a waxing.

Now don't get me wrong; the treatments I do are still medical procedures. They are safer, they are faster, and they are better than the procedures of the generation before—but they still are medical procedures that carry small degrees of risk. I'm thrilled that society is taking more comfort and acceptance of these procedures. But as you'll read about in this book, they are not benign. You just need to be a smart consumer about where to go and who should be taking care of your cosmetic needs.

Appreciating that you have the health and drive to engage in self-care is a luxury of life. It's a blessing to be able to have treatments that will make you look and feel good. This, in and of itself, will dramatically up that satisfaction potential. If you and those you love are healthy, safe, and have the basics essentials of life covered, you are playing with the house's money.

It's unfortunate that the words "Botox," "filler," and "laser" still have a connotation of unnecessary vanity. Few know that Botox has several indications approved by the US Food and Drug Administration (FDA) to improve health, from muscle spasms to migraines. Using fillers to add volume to your face helps bring back the collagen and healthy connective tissue lost in middle age. Laser resurfacing doesn't just get rid of wrinkles—it decreases skin cancer risk by removing sun damage.

So many of my patients admit that they feel bad about spending money on cosmetic treatments. They feel bad about being concerned about their appearance. I reassure them that they deserve to treat themselves now, because there will come a time in everyone's life where their looks will be the least of their worries. I spend a lot of time with these patients debunking the stigma about taking care of your appearance, because the essence of pro-aging is that treating the outside leads to changes on the inside—and vice versa.

One of the myths is that if you do things to look youthful, you're putting yourself at significant risk. Another is that all cosmetic procedures are going to end up looking fake. And the classic stereotype about people who go to cosmetic dermatologists (and cosmetic surgeons) is that they're crazy and vain. That they're ladies with disposable income and too much time on their hands. That they're gay men obsessed with their looks. That they are obsessive about turning back the clock and want to look as young as possible at any cost.

That is just not true. My patients range in age from their twenties to their nineties, almost half and half men and women, all quite different but with one thing in common: they want to be the best versions of themselves. I love meeting the unexpected patient, like the burly Harley-Davidson type who comes to me for love-handle liposuction, or the quiet librarian type who wants a little filler in her lip. Because everybody looks in the mirror with aspirations, and everyone likes results.

My patients are getting younger all the time; the largest growth in my practice is from those who are twenty-five to thirty-five. Nearly all of the new devices and new drugs are being created for early stage aging. My patients are savvy enough to start young. They know that it's much easier to clean your room when it's not dirty, and that when you do start early, you don't need as much help later on.

Furthermore, many of these patients, especially the younger ones, are not wealthy at all; they save up for the treatments they want. With all the amazing advances in dermatology—not just in my office but also available over the counter—there's something out there for everyone's price point. Something that actually works!

Still, I'm not a plastic surgeon. Plastic surgeons can change people. I don't—I *optimize*. Occasionally, to be sure, I give people lips that they never had, or more defined cheekbones, or a different arch of their eyebrows, but, in general, what I do maximizes what my patients have already. I always say that everybody wants to look good simply fitting back into their jeans and t-shirts like when they were younger. With laser resurfacing, I want to get women back to the time when makeup enhanced their features rather than covered imperfections.

Pro-aging is about rejuvenation, *not reinvention.*

Pro-aging is about *rejuvenation*, not reinvention. My goal is to pro-age you gracefully. When people take good care of themselves, you don't know their age. You just know they exude vitality and confidence. That's what makes them beautiful.

Age Is Just a Number

There's so much ageism in the beauty and wellness business that it's the elephant in the room—because too many people still associate beauty with youth.

What most patients want as they grow older is not the fountain of youth. Of course, everybody wants to look a little younger and more noticeable, but they also want to look *vital* and healthy, like the lovely ninety-four-year old patient I mentioned earlier.

Unfortunately, as you get older, natural alterations of your anatomy take place, and these can make you look sad, angry, unhealthy, exhausted, and/or saggy. These visual interpretations have emotional ramifications for those around you. Patients tell me that everyone is asking them why they are so tired or angry when they're neither. This is enough to make them feel tired and angry! It's why I believe Botox may well be FDA-approved for depression—really, it's happening! Because when you look angry and tired due to your wrinkles, and then Botox makes your wrinkles go away, then you *do* feel less angry and tired. There have been so many psychological studies about how looking better makes you feel better. It's just our nature. And I think that is where ageism comes into play.

Most people, including my seventy-eight-year-old father, still feel thirty years old inside. At fifty, I'm certainly starting to be far more aware of my own aging than I was a few years ago. As well as I take care of myself and as good as I look, there's a misalignment sometimes. Some mornings are better than others. Pro-aging is about having more of those good days.

I can't change who you are. Everyone has a good face, that version of themselves in a certain photograph at a certain angle where they look their best. If you come to see me, my job is to give you more of that. If you do it on your own, with this book, your job is to give *you* more of that—physically and emotionally. Because if you're miserable, it doesn't matter how many treatments you have. You're still going to be miserable.

That's what pro-aging is all about.

Pro-Aging from the Inside Out and the Outside In

Henry is a longtime patient in his early fifties. He always rushed in, slightly disgruntled that he had to have any treatments, while admitting they were an important part of his competitiveness at work to stay youthful and appear vital. I sensed his subtle level of dissatisfaction because I knew his heart wasn't in it. His sense of self was tied into the way he looked, and he felt it affected his job and his lifestyle and relationships. He was burning the candle at both ends and basically just frustrated with life. Even though he kept coming back and respected my skills—injectable treatments and a little bit of laser every time—he was always slightly dissatisfied, looking for a quicker fix or a better answer.

At one point, six months went by before his next visit, and I noticed he'd lost a significant amount of weight. After I complimented him, he said, "You know, I had to take stock of my life and change my priorities. I changed how I ate. I started meditating and exercising more. Doing the things you and others I respect had mentioned." He finally took the time to fully deal with his own well-being rather than the exterior things he thought would make him happy.

I knew that Henry hadn't made these changes because of me—he knew he had to take better care of himself—but he had reached that crucial tipping point. We had a great talk, and I gave him the same treatments I had performed over the years. A few weeks later, he sent me a note telling me how amazing everything had turned out this time, for the first time. I called him right away and said, "I did everything *exactly* the same, you know. *You're* the reason why the treatments are so much better. You lost weight and you empowered yourself at the gym and you prioritized yourself, which made other aspects of your life better. You obviously changed things about your work and your life habits and you're looking at things differently. You are now pro-aging, and my treatments are just the icing on the cake."

Henry had learned that happiness and positivity can't be injected. Every time he comes to see me now, he feels stronger and more comfortable in his own skin. He is now a better version of himself.

People who look and feel good know that beauty and health are the *same*. Lots of things we do for our health make us look good, and lots of things we can do to our skin to look good will actually make our skin healthier.

Which brings me to the notion of success. As I said, you can't just do one thing. People take for granted what success is, personally or professionally, and it's something that excuses are often made for. What many don't realize is that "overnight sensations" are decades in the making. Sure, there are strikes of lightning, both positive and negative, for some people in this world—but most personal and professional success is a hard grind of habit forming, overcoming innumerous challenges, and developing clearly defined thought processes that require ceaseless focus. It can't be bought, and it ain't luck. Whether you're Michael Jordan or Steve Jobs or even the Kardashians, there needs to be vision, intent, discipline, and sacrifice for achievement.

This is also true about ourselves in achieving happiness, a feeling of beauty, and professional and emotional purpose. We often like to make excuses for other people's success and happiness...that a shortcut or favor was bestowed, that it was a fluke of timing, or that a genetic mutation allowed the individual to achieve greatness. Well, we certainly don't live in a universe where all things are created equal, but you can bet, when you meet someone who's successful at life, that it's not a coincidence, and that it's often a result of self-care and the manifestation of goal-oriented conduct.

Most people are searching for something to better their lives—an answer, a pill, a shot, a diet, a routine, a secret weapon, a shortcut. Let me put you at ease: There is no shortcut and there is no one answer. Feeling well, looking good, thinking positively, and being vital takes effort as we age. No one just rolls out of bed happy and content—not at any age! That doesn't mean we don't continue our search and stay open-minded to new pathways to success. But everything has checks and balances, particularly drugs and procedures; there is no sweet without some sour. All choices have consequences, good and bad.

With open-mindedness and discipline, there is going to be a journey where you're going to find your ideal balance. If you want to feel good, think positively, and look good, that's going to take work. Anything in life worth having takes work. Because then you have the satisfaction of setting goals and reaching them. And when you achieve those goals, you set the bar a little higher and move on to the next goals. Finding and experimenting with what fits for you...that is the embraceable journey—and that is where pro-aging begins.

Realize too that once professional and personal goals are achieved, smooth sailing is *not* a given. Despite the spoils and advantages that success brings, it's often more difficult to stay on top. This reminds me of quote by Jonas Salk, developer of the polio vaccine: "The reward for work well done is the opportunity to do well." The hill climbed often becomes steeper toward the top, with forces and people to pull you down.

Pro-aging is about developing an attitude that recognizes what personal and professional success requires. It's about remaining adaptable and innovative once goals are achieved in any aspect of life—this is what keeps us all going. It is the food for vitality! I have patients who can't stand their aging eyes and don't want surgery, so I do what I can cosmetically to improve their situation and then tell them to get some funky glasses they'll love to wear. When you recognize, appreciate, and work toward what it takes to get to your goals and to stay there, you'll find the spoils of personal, aesthetic, and professional success come quite easily.

My mentors that I find motivational inspire me to be the best version of myself, just as my family inspires me to be part of my community. People tell me they want to grow old gracefully, yet they don't want to put in any effort. There's actually nothing graceful about that because it's hard work to grow old. "Old age ain't no place for sissies," said Bette Davis. There's nothing graceful about the progressive decrepitude of the human body. And I don't just mean the way you look. I mean that if you don't take care of yourself, you age very quickly. I think we're spoiled by modern medicine. If you go to third-world countries where people don't have access to healthcare, people die much younger. Growing old gracefully is more about working as hard as you can to stay healthy, feel healthy, and look healthy.

Adapt, adjust, own it. That is pro-aging.

Let me show you how to find the balance for yourself—and become a pro-aging pro.

PART ONE

NOURISH YOUR OUTSIDE

CHAPTER 1

Over-the-Counter Skin Care

Confidence breeds beauty.

—ESTÉE LAUDER

Using the best skincare products for you is an important part of your pro-aging protocol, but I have to admit that discussing them is one of more frustrating skincare topics. Why? Because there is already so much information out there—most of which is either wrong or drenched in hype, full of misconceptions and fear-mongering about what does and doesn't work.

This is where the complexities of over-the-counter (OTC) skincare products come into play. There's an enormous amount of products on the market "to help battle signs of aging." There are firming gels, tightening serums, antipollution products, collagen stimulators, hormone regulators, retinoids, wrinkle smoothers, skin lighteners and brighteners—you name it. I could write a ten-volume encyclopedia on all these items, active ingredients, and inactive ingredients and whether or not they actually work. If you are a typical skincare-product shopper, you've already been bombarded with cosmetic companies gushing praise and market-ing strategies for the newest and the trendiest and the most-touted products, most of which will be obsolete a few months later.

> *With products, less is often more.* Protect your skin, but don't treat it—*especially when little to nothing is* wrong *with it.*

While it's great to have so many choices, and excellent prod-ucts abound, succumbing to the lure of tempting new products with splashy ad campaigns and influencer endorsements is not the point of pro-aging. I don't want to tell you what to use. I want to tell you what to *avoid*.

My contrarian point of view is that, with products, less is often more. This means the most important step of all is to *protect your skin*. Don't treat your skin, especially when little to nothing is wrong with it. This is where the pro in *pro*active comes in—because you don't need most of these hyped-up products.

Enjoy your self-care. Taking care of your skin shouldn't be seen as a chore. It's not about dutifully putting on anti-aging creams or sunscreen, or using eight different products twice a day because you feel you have to, so there's no reason why your daily rituals can't be pleasurable. If you love being a product junkie, so be it—load up. Just keep it simple!

> *Enjoy your self-care. Taking care of your skin shouldn't be seen as a chore.*

Skin Basics

Once you know the basics about your body's largest organ, you'll be better able to determine which skincare claims are legit and which are bogus.

There is no single cause of aging, and the battle of nature versus nurture is one that will never have a clear winner. Both our genetics and our environment play very significant roles, and there will always be variations and predispositions in every aspect of health. Some people never go gray, for example, while others suffer hair loss in their thirties. Some have oily skin and few wrinkles, and others have such pronounced frown lines that people think they are perpetually angry when they're not.

Although there are countless variations in skin color and tone, skin itself is basically the same for everyone. Its job is to respond to the environment, to prevent water loss, and to maintain body-heat regulation—in other words, to protect, to regulate, and to metabolize. Its biological functions don't necessarily have to do with what you see in the mirror. If you keep challenging it, damaging it, either with extremes of weather and sun or topical drugs or the wrong skincare products, the evidence will be very visible.

Skin Anatomy

Your skin is comprised of three major layers: the epidermis on top, the dermis, and the bottom layer, or the subcutis (also known as the fat layer).

The epidermis has five of its own layers: The topmost, called the stratum corneum, is made up of dead skin cells that protect the layers beneath. (Yes, dead skin has a valuable, necessary function.) They slough off naturally every two to four weeks, but as you get older, this shedding takes longer—up to two months! Which is why your skin can look dull, unless it is regularly exfoliated. And the epidermis also contains melanin-rich melanocytes, the skin cells responsible for skin's pigmentation.

The dermis is the structural layer that contains keratinocytes, the machines of collagen and elastin, the protein fibers that give your skin elasticity, firmness, and resilience. It also contains hyaluronic acid, which holds in moisture, among other connective tissue components, glands, and hair follicles.

The subcutis is your skin's fatty, protective, and cushioning layer, rich with blood vessels, oil glands, and nerves. The oil produced by these glands pushes its way up to the surface via your pores, and keeps your skin hydrated and protected from the inside. Fat has several biologic functions, including hormone production and regulation, and it is necessary for survival.

Intrinsic and Extrinsic Aging

As we get older, changes in our skin are inevitable.

- **Intrinsic aging** is due to factors you can't control: your genetic predisposition to wrinkles in certain areas, oil content that might be high when you're young and far lower as you get older, the slowing rate of skin-cell turnover, acne, pigmentation changes, the normal loss of collagen and elastin (which leads to sagging and wrinkles), and hormonal changes, especially lower levels of estrogen and testosterone, as we age.

- **Extrinsic aging** is due to factors over which you have more control: sun exposure, weather exposure, pollution, sleep deprivation, a suboptimal diet, smoking, excessive drinking and drug use, and, of course, stress. When you're overwhelmed, it's going to show on your skin!

Skincare Basics

Whenever I'm asked what people should do for their skin care, I always say, "What bothers you? *That's* what you need to take care of." A person with acne will have different needs than someone with hyperpigmentation spots; a person with oily skin will not want super rich emollients the way someone with very dry and sun-damaged skin will.

Unless you have specific skincare problems, however, I will repeat my mantra: *Protect your skin—don't treat it.*

I've seen patients who went to college in Arizona or Florida, and by the time they're twenty-five, a road map has already been etched into their skin. Others who grow up in cloudy and freezing Michigan or Minnesota have little sun damage. Many who are African-American or Indian or Asian don't show signs of aging until much later. Everyone's skin is unique—but everyone can benefit from becoming a skincare minimalist.

Which is why, when my patients bring in their overloaded bag full of the beauty products they use on a daily basis, they're absolutely shocked that I barely look through it. Instead, I push my foot on the pedal and drop the entire bag in the garbage. "Time to subtract, not add," I tell them. Why? Because, as you'll see in the section on sensitive skin syndrome on page 20, overuse of products is one of the primary causes of messed-up skin. Using different layers of different products can not only cause intense irritation, but counteract each other, rendering them basically useless—especially if you're not participating in the simple tasks of minimizing and managing the extrinsic factors that are aging your skin.

When your skin is in decent shape, all you need to do is use a simple cleanser, sunscreen, and moisturizer. That's the basic minimum and can often be enough. If you want to add a product, do it one at a time. It's totally fine to use it for a long time. Everyone loves to tell the story of their elder relative who looks great and only uses Nivea or Noxzema cold cream. Actually, it wasn't the product that did the trick—it was the simplicity and the consistency...the focus on using that product faithfully, rather than the constant distraction of other options.

> *The best product will always be the one that works for your skin and fits into your budget. As with everything in life, if it suits you and you put faith in it, then it will serve you well.*

As there are so many components in OTC skincare products, it's an individual decision to find the right ones. There are active ingredients you might like, even if they aren't as strong as prescription medications (like retinol, which is a weaker version of prescription-only Tretinoin). There are different scents and textures you might prefer. There is packaging. All of these options are valid ones, and if you like a super-expensive cream that makes your skin smooth and smell divine, and you can afford it, go for it. Just realize that price often has much more to do with hype, packaging, and marketing than the quality of the ingredients. Fantastic products don't have to be expensive. The best product will always be the one that works for your skin and fits into your budget. As with everything in life, if it suits you and you put faith in it, then it will serve you well.

Active and Inactive Ingredients

Skincare products have active and inactive ingredients.

Active ingredients are the ones that are theoretically going to have a biologic effect on the skin, for your benefit. If an active ingredient is considered a drug, it must be listed separately in a box labeled Drug Facts/Active Ingredients on the packaging.

Inactive ingredients are all of the various things that are going to help keep the products on the shelf without contamination, such as preservatives. They are also what affects the texture and the scent—the sensory and absorption components of the formulation to give you a comfortable experience and deliver the active ingredients.

Consumers usually choose a product based on the active ingredients, but something you likely don't know is that the *inactive* ingredients—the formulation itself—are almost always the reason why you like or can tolerate a product. You could have something with an effective active ingredient like retinol or vitamin C, but if the scent or the texture isn't appealing or if it causes irritation, you won't like it or use it.

In addition, certain active ingredients should never be used together. If you like a vitamin A (retinol) serum and add a moisturizer with vitamin C, for example, this seemingly benign and "healthy" combination can make your skin supersensitive and susceptible to damage.

Always read the labels before buying any skincare product. You'll likely see a long list of unpronounceable chemicals, most of which are completely benign, and if you're worried about any of them, look them up. Cyclopentasiloxane, for instance, sounds scary, but it's just a synthetic silicone used in sunscreen and hair products as a lubricant. Doing a few minutes of research will also direct you to legit sites that assess the effectiveness and/or potential toxicity and side effects of these ingredients.

Over-Hyped Ingredients

In order for an OTC product to work effectively, it needs to contain active ingredients (such as retinol or vitamin C) that can penetrate into your skin. Many skincare companies tout ingredients that can't really do that.

Most consumers don't know this. Instead, they rely on the hype, ads, articles, social media postings, and word of mouth to make skincare choices. You'll see the word "may" a lot, as in "This cream may improve wrinkles." Or, "Over 90 percent saw visible improvements!" Well, how many people were in that 90 percent testing group? Five, twenty, two thousand? How was the testing done? The efficacy level is not going to appear on the packaging. The fact that collagen is an ingredient doesn't mean it can actually affect your existing collagen—because it can't penetrate into your skin; seeing that plant stem cells are in a cream doesn't mean that they will have a biologic absorption and effect.

It's important to be aware of clever marketing that disguises the fact that the "new new" is really just the "old old," with different packaging or a reformulated texture. Companies often make drug-like claims for items that aren't drugs. Ignore the hype. The beauty business is unbelievably competitive, and it's extremely difficult to not only make a difference but make a profit. Hence, the sometimes outrageous claims.

Remember my mantra: Protect your skin first—treat second. Avoid self-diagnosis and see a dermatologist if you have a condition that doesn't improve or is new (like a sudden onset of acne, which is often hormone-related, or a mole changing in any way). Often, skin issues arise from the products you may be using, so talk to a professional.

Is "All-Natural" Bogus?

Two of the most often abused and misused words you can see on any packaging, whether for food or cosmetics, are "all natural."

The entire world we live in is all natural. Nourishing plants are all natural. Plague, disease, storms, botulism, poison ivy, snake venom, and cocaine are all natural too. There is a false perception that "all natural" is all good. The fact of the matter is: the reason why we're alive and have the longevity we do is because we've developed things to battle the all-natural in nature. Every great medicine is derived from all-natural compounds that we use for healing, but curative purposes can also be toxic if used improperly or in large doses. Although there may be synthetic chemicals in the world that may be harmful, there is an enormous amount of human innovation in synthetic goods that provide great value and safety to the world.

Natural beauty is also confused and aligned with "clean" beauty. Clean beauty can be synthetic or natural but gives the connotation that it is universally safe, not harmful, and often has an eco-friendly footprint. Sadly, there is no standard or gauge or committee that monitors the stamp of "clean" beauty, so the phrase is heavily abused by marketing specialists.

We all want products that are universally safe, that work, that last on shelves, that smell great, that can be used by everyone, and that are eco-friendly and affordable. Well, world peace is also an ideal goal. Educate yourself, experiment, and just be cautious about the verbal marketing ploys of the products out there. Consumers want to feel good about their products, and companies that care most about profits take advantage of that.

Organic Skincare Products

The only way you can ascertain if a product is legitimately organic is if it has received Certified Organic approval from the USDA. As you can see from the list of prohibited and allowed items for organic plants and animals listed at www.ecfr.gov, it is extremely difficult and costly to become certified. This is why organic products tend to be pricier than nonorganic.

Companies that follow the regulations to be certified organic will have a seal on their packaging that says "USDA Organic." That means the product must contain at least 95 percent organic ingredients. Any item that says "Made with Organic Ingredients" has to contain at least 70 percent organic ingredients. Any item that just says "Organic," which some skincare products do if even a tiny amount of a certain ingredient is organic, is likely a rip-off if you're seeking a fully organic item.

The Preservatives Debate

Skincare products need to contain chemical preservatives in order to have a long shelf life. Without them, your creams could become contaminated with dangerous bacteria and putrid within a matter of weeks. Or less. Preservative-free is not an automatic plus when buying products. Most people don't know that the most commonly used preservatives have been around for decades, have been extensively tested, and are generally safe for human use. Some preservatives are better than others, of course, but, from a doctor's standpoint, preservative-free claims will never entice me to buy a product.

PABA and Parabens

Certain ingredients get an undeserved, universal bad rap only because a very small group of people had a problem with them.

In the early days of sunscreen formulation, PABA (para-aminobenzoic acid) was commonly used in sunscreens. A certain percentage of people were allergic, had reactions, became vocal, and this created so much negative hype that current sunscreens are almost always PABA-free. For the skin technology of the time, PABA was an effective agent. The same thing happened with aluminum chlorohydrate, an ingredient in antiperspirants that was allegedly accused of causing breast cancer, despite many studies proving it did not. This created negative media hype and what some believe was unfounded pressure to take it out of formulas.

Parabens met the same fate, although they've historically been one of the best, safest, and most cost-effective preservatives to prevent bacteria from spoiling a product. They're an amazing stabilizer.

Should those with allergies or reactions to skincare ingredients be discounted? Of course not. But what is the tipping point for deciding to yank an ingredient or not? As with PABA, a very small percentage of people had reactions to parabens, which morphed into an erroneous assumption that parabens were not only toxic but hormone disrupters and carcinogenic. This negative hype keeps people away from ingredients that could be potentially useful.

Yet most people don't know what you just read about parabens, and that I believe the hype about not using them is overblown. We live in a world where the ill-informed are screaming not only about the dangers of parabens, but about the dangers of safe and effective vaccines, which literally puts millions of vulnerable people at risk for serious illness and even death. This doesn't mean that I want to bathe my body in aluminum chlorohydrate or overexpose myself to products with parabens every single day. There are small risks to everything. But I'm talking about moderate use for specific reasons.

There's no question in my mind that preservatives like parabens have proven to increase the safety and the shelf life of skincare products. Are there better alternatives? Doubtless there will be, and we should work toward creating them. This is part of the reason why I believe everything should be minimal or, at most, used in moderation. Nothing is universally good for you! Just because a drug may have the potential to cause harm when used *inappropriately* doesn't mean the *appropriate* dosage can't be safe and effective. So am I concerned about putting limited amounts of parabens on my skin? I am not. No convincing data to date has convinced me that they pose a significant health threat when used in moderation. It's a point of contention, but I'm allowed my opinion too!

Everything is about balance, whether food, skincare, or chemicals. You can't demonize or aggrandize anything too much or too little. We wouldn't be alive if not for vaccines or preservatives. That doesn't mean we don't have to hold the pharmaceutical industry to the highest standards to prove product efficacy. That doesn't mean that an extremely small number of people can't have bad reactions to vaccines. But there is no legit scientist in the world who would say that the longevity and wellness of mankind have not been improved by vaccinations.

Once again, do your homework. If something concerns you, read the science—not the opinions. Talk to a dermatologist. If you have any doubts about any ingredient, you can always find a product that contains those you deem safe. There are many affordable options.

The Fragrance Debate

Another hot topic is fragrance-free products. As with any ingredient, a small minority of people are allergic or sensitive to fragrance. They respond to it by itchy red rashes or just plain irritation. Unfortunately, it's often impossible to pinpoint what precisely is causing the reaction, because fragrance is always listed as just "fragrance" on the label, so you can't know what exactly its true composition is. The FDA allows the general terminology to be used as a group of various chemicals. This list can include up to five thousand molecules that are commonly used in heavy rotation in the skincare industry. The FDA exempts these products from having to be more specific, even though they might contain synthetic, preservative, or allergy-provoking substances that you might want to know about.

Yet the demand for fragrance-free has permeated the beauty industry, and it's a bit of a fallacy. "Fragrance-free" does not mean totally devoid of scent. It just means *fragrance*-free. Many fragrance-free products have natural, plant-based, or chemical masking scents in them to disguise the unpleasant odor of their chemical ingredients. Without these masking agents, the products would stink.

Part of the skincare experience is your nose. If we went totally fragrance-free in our lives, we would be very smelly people. Why do you think perfume became so popular before the medical advances of the twentieth century? Because without deodorant, good hygiene, indoor plumbing, and regular bathing, people reeked unless they doused themselves, their wigs, their clothing, their fans, and their handkerchiefs with perfume.

So if you're worried about fragrance allergies or irritations, consult an allergist who can test you. You can focus your attention on more natural, flower- and plant-based essential oils and scents that may be better for you. But realize that these too can pose similar problems. Trial and error, people. Trial and error!

Give Your Products a Chance to Work, and That Means One at a Time

Active ingredients take weeks to work. You're *never* going to see a difference overnight. If you do, it's because of the inactive ingredients that cause a nonbiologic "appearance" to the skin, like a form of makeup.

I tell everyone that unless you have bad reaction to a new product, you must always use it for at least four to six *weeks* before you can assess any real results. In that regard, skincare products are no different than oral medications. When you start taking a prescription medication, such as one to treat high blood pressure or an antidepressant, your doctor will want to see you a month or six weeks later to assess not only if it is working, but also if you are tolerating the medicine. Any new medicine can take time to adjust to, with or without side effects. That's because drugs need to be metabolized over time to reach therapeutic levels in your body and be given time to have a clinical effect.

If products are selling you an immediate result, realize this often has to do with the *inactive* ingredients, such as mica or silicone, that give you a sheen and/or brighten your skin as they reflect light. They're there only to give you reinforcement to allow the active ingredients to take hold in your skin. Active ingredients *always* take a few weeks to become really effective.

In addition, if you add more than one new product to your regimen, you won't know what works, or what could be causing problems. If, however, you're going to the dermatologist and are given a regimen of two or three products, don't worry. Your doctor has already assessed your skin and knows what should be helpful in combination.

Bottom line: There's no way to make a long-term biologic difference of anti-wrinkle or firming results in the skin in a couple of days. If a laser takes time, if Botox takes time, if everything else takes time to see the results, what do you think a cream is going to do?

Hopefully, knowing this will save you not only potential skin irritation, but money, because it's way too easy to try a new product, not see any changes in a week or two, think it's no good, chuck it, and buy something else. Many products too need adjustments. Retinoids and antioxidant products like retinol, both prescription and OTC, can cause irritation. Sometimes, you have to see if your skin adjusts and tolerates it. Or even start using it slowly a few times a week. Point being, give it a chance. You might be pleasantly surprised that something you thought didn't work is actually the perfect product for you.

New Is Not Always Better

Something I tell patients over and over is that I want to help them find a skincare product that works for them that they will stick with forever. Everyone's got the hot new product—but new is not always better. Find your brand loyalty and stick with it.

I spent several years as a brand ambassador for Estée Lauder, and I worked on several of their product lines. They have patents on a multitude of different ingredients, and they, like many skin-care companies, use some of the same ingredients in several of their product lines. The differences in these lines may be in the inactive ingredients, packaging, marketing, publicity, and various formulation tweaks. Sometimes, older active ingredients are used in a hot new product—because they were known to be effective—but there were enough small changes to make the product seem completely different. Was this new product *better*? Topically, maybe, if you liked the scent and packaging of it, or it felt lovely as you applied it, or you liked the story of the brand or its ethos. The product may serve you in some way, but the cosmetic result of the product may not be better.

There's also a luxury placebo effect. I have to confess that I'm susceptible to it. I sometimes buy a new perfume or product because the bottle is so enticing or the packaging is so attractive. Does that make these items *better*? No, it just makes them more desirable to my sensibility! It serves me, which I guess is good enough.

When the skincare products my patients use remain effective, I don't want to start switching things up. If changes are needed, I usually go back to basics, erase everything, then add things one at a time. And, of course, give them time to work.

The Difference Between Big Companies and Small Companies

One thing patients often ask me about is whether they should avoid products from large skincare conglomerates and opt for those of smaller companies. Since I've had the opportunity to work with brands on both ends of the spectrum and in between, I can say that the answer might be different than what you'd expect.

Regulations are very stringent for skincare companies. They have to abide by an enormous regulatory board, both legally, in terms of what their medical claims are, and with the testing of their products.

There's an automatic reflex to be fearful of big industry, especially big pharma. But I can tell you from my personal experience with large skincare companies that, thanks to their resources and their need to abide by regulatory requirements, both legally and safety-wise, they are forced to dot their i's and cross their t's. They're also regulated by the consumers' watchful eye to make sure there's no animal testing, among other travesties. Big companies such as Estée Lauder do big business with a huge global audience; if they do not do their due diligence and follow the rules, there will be trouble.

My biggest concern—and there are exceptions to every rule—is that smaller companies struggle with their profit margins in such a saturated and competitive industry. They don't have the money for the research and development and the elaborate product safety testing required. They don't have the population to test the products on. And they don't have the large audience either. As with the supplement industry, many of these smaller companies don't necessarily reveal all of their active testing, or all of their active or inactive ingredients. Everyone loves the small-brand story, its authenticity, its grassroots approach to finding untapped niches. But often, small companies fly under the radar and avoid stringent regulatory responsibilities in several aspects of their product development, their legal claims, and their efficacy.

As a result, and certainly with exception, I feel more comfortable recommending products from big companies. Their products might not always live up to the hype, but they are more likely to be safe, have intense research and development behind them, and be stringently tested. That doesn't mean there aren't incredible products made by smaller companies. It's just up to you to be a smart consumer and find them. Don't always fall for the unicorn.

Over-the-Counter Products

You're Probably Cleansing Your Face All Wrong

When you protect your body and allow it to do its job, you'd be shocked at how well it will take care of you.

Overzealous cleansing and exfoliating strip the skin of its natural protective oils. Many people overdo it.

As you learned earlier, the stratum corneum—the dead-skin-cell layer of your epidermis—helps maintain body temperature and hydration levels. It contains a thin, slightly acidic film called the acid mantle. The acid mantle is made up of natural oils, sweat, and sebum, which prevent harmful (naturally alkaline) contaminants from damaging the skin. When you strip too much of this layer, either through excessive washing or exfoliation, it will become irritated and susceptible to damage and infection. The acid mantle is also protective against bacteria, environmental pollutants, and moisture loss.

I get frustrated by the mania for super "clean" and constant exfoliation. It's not needed because the stratum corneum, aka your topmost dead-skin layer, has a true protective biologic function and should not be removed completely. Most dermatologists would warn against over-exfoliation, but many, not all, aestheticians like to exfoliate because it reinforces their job and they make money by selling products. As we age, yes, we need to exfoliate a bit more often for slowing cell turnover. But it's far more common that people overdo this process rather than ignore it.

There is a role in your pro-aging regimen for mild to moderate exfoliation, since skin-cell turnover slows with age and can leave your complexion looking dull. But certainly not twice a day, every day. Not with harsh exfoliants either. Don't forget that cleansing itself, especially if you use a washcloth, is a physical exfoliation as well. Some people are using a cleanser, a scrub, *and* a toner. Men, in addition, are actively exfoliating by shaving. All these habits can contribute to sensitive skin syndrome, which you'll read about in the next section, and can often be avoided.

All you need to do is clean your face twice a day, especially in the evening, if you wear makeup. If you are running late in the morning, or if your skin is super dry, gently clean your face just with water. Be sure to use a cleanser at night to get rid of the grime of the day before bed. Do you need multiple steps? Absolutely not!

People also think acne is caused by dirty skin or eating greasy foods, which it's not. It's most often caused by genetics and hormones, the *p. acnes* bacteria, and exacerbated by stress, lack of sleep, lack of exercise, and eating way too much of inflammation-producing items like sugar, processed foods, and dairy products. Over-cleansing acne can actually make it worse, as this triggers skin to produce *more* oil, leading to more clogged pores and blemishes.

A little dirt is not a bad thing. We're learning more and more that the immune system needs to be challenged at an early age, and that too much cleaning in too sterile of an environment can have serious health repercussions, like allergies and asthma, later in life. That's why people who grow up outdoors tend to be healthier—not just because they're more physically active than city-dwellers, but because they have their hands in dirt all day long!

Sensitive Skin Syndrome

The average American woman uses five to ten new products every year, and that number is going up. In Asia, skin care is far more regimented. In South Korea, the average man uses *seven* different products on his daily regimen. And women use up to fifteen. *Fifteen!*

All is well and good if there are no associated skin problems, but frequent in-office skin complaints come from one major, common issue: using too many products.

Sensitive skin syndrome is a clinical malady that causes your skin to react to everything you put on it. Nothing seems to be working for you, no matter what you do. Ironically, in most cases, this is the result of an overuse of too many products, too much manipulation over a short period of time, or sensitivities you have developed to certain ingredients. It's your body saying that it's tired of having itself challenged by various products. We have to give pause, we have to let your skin heal, we have to not challenge it, maybe get allergy-tested, and we have to start from scratch. The goal is to keep things simple.

If you have sensitive skin syndrome, go back to basics: clean, protect, and hydrate. That's it. Cleanser, sunscreen, and moisturizer. Give Dove Beauty Bar a try again. The Dove bars are moisturizing, not really a soap, and they won't stress your skin (or your pocketbook!). Be wary of liquid soaps for your face, as the ingredients that make them liquefied can be irritating. Once the sensitized skin has normalized, with or without the help of a dermatologist, you can slowly add products back, one at a time, or just keep it simple. You may just find out what the original culprit was that caused the problem.

Hydration and Moisturizer Basics

The Hydration You Need

Next time you're tempted to spend a lot of money on the newest moisturizer with the sumptuous texture and gorgeous packaging, remember that outer and inner hydration are not mutually exclusive. Most people think about hydration from the outside, but you should also be getting it from within. You can put all the moisture on that you want, but if you don't stay hydrated and well-nourished thanks to what you eat and drink, the biological functions of your cells aren't going to absorb the external moisture very well. Slathering on the serums and creams is a waste of time and money, unless you're properly hydrated and fed from the inside.

How much should you hydrate yourself internally every day? That depends on your activity level, and how much you exercise and sweat. For most people, this is six to eight glasses of water a day. The basic rule is that if your urine is clear and white, you're well-hydrated. If it's yellow, you're either dehydrated or you're taking a lot of vitamins. Because that's where most vitamins go: out of your wallet, into your mouth, and into your urine! But more on that later.

The Moisturizers You Need

As you know, your skin is a highly metabolic, very sophisticated organ whose job is to protect itself. It's the gatekeeper for all things in and out—not just moisture, but heat and toxins. It is constantly variable, depending on the weather, other elements, hormones, and genetics. For most people, some areas of their skin will need more moisturizing than others, especially as we get older and there is less oil production. It's perfectly fine to use two different moisturizers, one richer or not, on different parts of the face as needed.

Most moisturizers are a mix of oil, water, and molecules, such as hyaluronic acid (a natural polysaccharide found in skin), that help draw in fluid. To be most effective and provide moisture from the outside, a moisturizer has to be able to break that natural skin barrier so that it is truly absorbed within. Hyaluronic acid draws water into the skin, but many other over-hyped ingredients may not. That includes oils. It's not quite true that putting oil on your skin provides a lot of moisture, because it can serve as a barrier on the surface and not get absorbed at all. It may just make your skin shiny.

Moisturizers come in different thicknesses:

- *Lotions* are the thinnest and the least hydrating and go on the skin very easily.
- *Gels* are medium thick and generally better for oilier skin.
- *Creams* are generally richer.

Ointments, such as Vaseline, are the thickest, with the highest concentration of oil. This can cause breakouts as they are occlusive and can clog pores, but they're also therapeutic for those with skin diseases such as eczema or psoriasis, or just extremely dry skin.

Serums are usually treatment products. They might contain ingredients like hyaluronic acid that help retain moisture, and most often target aspects of aging. They're an add-on to your regular, simple regimen of cleansing/sun protection/moisturizing, and you don't need them if your skin is normal and you don't want or need to target anything specific.

For some common serums, look for these active ingredients:

- Retinols, which help with fine lines and wrinkles, and collagen building.
- Peptides, which improve elasticity and skin tightening by helping with the development of proteins and collagen in the skin.
- Basic amino acids, the building blocks of proteins, which can affect the way muscles contract as well as the texture of the skin.
- Antioxidants like vitamin C and many plant-based ingredients like resveratrol that help with cellular damage.

Growth factors that are either bioengineered or sourced from human or plant cells enhance maturation and communication between skin cells and may contribute to a more youthful appearance.

As with all skincare products, you're not going to know what moisturizer works long term on your skin until you try it for at least a few weeks. Choose one that feels good, smells good, doesn't cause you to break out, and doesn't break the bank. No moisturizer should cost a fortune. The ingredients are not necessarily expensive. The hype is.

Remember: no over-the-counter cream is ever capable of being as effective as a dermatologist's prescription medications or procedures. So if your skin needs help, go get it.

The Pro-Aging OTC Skincare Regimen

Your basic and essential pro-aging regimen is very easy: Clean, Protect, Hydrate. A few tips:

- Add new products one at a time.
- Give each one four to six weeks to expect results. See how well you tolerate it. If you experience any irritation or any other issues, discontinue use and start again with a different product.
- Use only products that you like! If you're not crazy about the scent or the texture or anything at all about your items, find something else. You're not going to want to use something that isn't pleasurable.

MORNING:

- Gently rinse face with just water or light cleanser.
- Apply moisturizer.
- Apply broad spectrum mineral sunscreen.

NIGHT:

- Wash with a gentle cleanser. Consider adding a toner if you had a lot of makeup on or any residue remains on your skin.
- Consider exfoliation two to three times a week with either a physical or chemical agent.
- Apply serum.
- Apply moisturizer.

Sunscreen Basics

When our parents' generation was growing up, their mothers and fathers would send them out to play, and when they saw redness, their parents would yell at them to come inside. That was their version of sunscreen. Or rather, sun-scream!

Back then, few people paid attention to the aftereffects of solar radiation, from sunburns and pigment spots to deadly melanoma. They didn't yet know the specifics about skin damage caused by UVA (ultraviolet-A) and UVB (ultraviolet-B) rays.

UVA is slightly less carcinogenic than UVB but actually more aging because it penetrates deeper into the skin to cause cellular damage over time. UVA is what's used in tanning booths, which is why I call them instant-aging booths. (Go in there with a wine cooler and a cigarette, and it's a great way to grow old quickly!) UVA is also able to pass through glass, which is why a lot of cars now have protective treatments on the windows.

UVB rays are what cause burns. In a controlled medical setting, however, UVB can be used to treat certain skin conditions, such as psoriasis and eczema.

SPF, or Sun Protection Factor, refers *only* to UVB, not UVA. A broad-spectrum sunscreen protects against both. Sunscreens can contain chemical blockers, physical blockers, or both.

Chemical Sunscreens

Chemical sunscreens, while effective against sunburn, contain various synthetic active ingredients. They work by absorbing UV rays and converting them into heat.

Although these chemicals work effectively to prevent sunburn, there are many problems and controversies with them. Over the past twenty years, studies have linked chemical sunscreens to low testosterone, altered sperm function, shorter pregnancies, disrupted birth weights, hormone disruption in men and women, traces of sunscreen in breast milk, and high rates of allergic skin rashes. They may be potentially carcinogenic, although there is no solid evidence as yet. They also cause irreparable harm to marine ecosystems, such as coral reefs, and will be regulated in Hawaii and possibly in Florida. This potential harm has finally hit the public consciousness, and even a large drugstore chain, CVS, will remove oxybenzone and octinoxate from their store-brand sunscreens under SPF 50 by the end of 2020.

No studies to date have been conclusive of the true long-term risk that chemical sunscreens pose to humans. We do know, however, that these chemicals can get absorbed into the bloodstream with daily use. When these chemical blockers were first released, they were touted as miracle workers (sound familiar?) that could prevent skin cancer. But now, they are yet another example of how potential negative long-term effects can't possibly be known when drugs are tested only for a short time before they're released to an unsuspecting public.

Chemical and Mineral Sunscreen Ingredients

Active Chemical Ingredients: Avobenzone (Parsol 1789), octinoxate, octisalate, octocrylene, oxybenzone, homosalate

Active Mineral Ingredients: Zinc oxide, titanium dioxide. (They've been the sole active ingredients in baby sunscreens for years due to their well-known safety profiles.)

Mineral (Physical) Sunscreens

Mineral sunscreens, or physical sunscreens, create a physical barrier on the top of your skin to prevent the harmful rays from penetrating inside. They reflect UVB rays and mostly reflect UVA rays, which can penetrate much deeper, making them the ideal choice for those with hyperpigmentation issues. They are the only sunscreens the FDA regards as generally safe and effective for daily use, as they have shown no evidence of hormone disruption and only very rarely cause any allergic reactions.

Which Sunscreen to Choose

Many sunscreens are combinations of chemical and mineral ingredients to make them more effective. You have to look at the Active Ingredients box on the label and see which ones are listed. Chemical sunscreens are still on the market because they work, they're inexpensive, they're cosmetically elegant, and they're easy to apply. When it comes to skin care, consumers don't just demand effective active ingredients, but ease of use. And people just love their sunscreen sprays.

The problem with mineral sunscreens has been that they weren't cosmetically elegant, meaning they were hard to apply and left white streaks everywhere. This made them especially unappealing to people of color. It was also difficult to put them into spray form. Luckily, one of the greatest recent breakthroughs in sunscreens is the reformulated and micronized versions of mineral blockers that apply more smoothly and are absorbed more rapidly.

I don't think there's much risk for adults who use chemical sunscreens occasionally during a vacation at the beach. But the problem is that parents slather chemical sunscreens all over the bodies of their babies and children at the beach several times a day, and these chemicals are absorbed into the bloodstream, leach into our water, are often inhaled in aerosols, and may cause harm to us and to the environment over time. This is why the American Pediatric Association recommends that only mineral sunscreen be used on babies and children. Many skincare companies are replacing chemical ingredients with natural alternatives as well. Read the labels before you buy any sunscreen!

Why People Who Use Sunscreen Still Get Skin Damage

Mineral sunscreens offer the best protection, and there's no question that, for children, they are the only sunscreen you should use. Some people use a combination, but we have to continue to improve the technology and the quality of sunscreens—and most important, we have to change the regulations. We cannot sell sun protection based on SPF alone, because it gives a false sense of security about sun protection. Putting on sunscreen in the morning is not enough. I've lost count of how many patients have come to see me with terrible sunburns for just that reason. Here's what you need to know:

- Underuse is one of the biggest problems with sunscreen. It's hard to apply it evenly and it's hard to apply enough. If you're going to be out in the sun for some time, you need to use a lot more sunscreen than you think you do. That means at least a tablespoon for your face and a few ounces for your body (a shot-glass-worth will do) in order to reach the full SPF level listed on the bottle. Using a spray is convenient, but apply it *inside*, ideally in a bathroom, then rub it in well; otherwise, it'll blow all over the place outside—everywhere but on your skin!

- You need to apply chemical sunscreen at least thirty minutes before going outside; mineral sunscreen works much quicker. Let it soak in for a few minutes and then rub it in again. If you're using moisturizer, put it on after sunscreen. (Bear in mind that, while many moisturizers contain SPF, people usually don't apply enough to get the full benefit of the SPF level. It's better to use a separate sunscreen and moisturizer if you have dry skin.) If you apply it only when you arrive at the beach, you're basically totally unprotected for thirty minutes.

- Always reapply sunscreen after swimming, after drying off, or if you've been sweating a lot. Otherwise, reapply every two hours.

- SPF measures potential burn time but only for UVB radiation, not UVA, which is another significant player in sun damage and aging. If it takes you ten minutes of unprotected sun to get a sunburn, SPF 30 will give you 300 minutes of protection before you start to burn. Everyone has a different burn rate, so to be safe rather than sorry, reapply every two hours. If this sounds confusing, it is. There is clearly room for greater regulatory control that simplifies the rating scales of protective sunscreen use.

- Use a product with an SPF 30 minimum that has either broad-spectrum coverage and/or UVB/UVA coverage. Anything above SPF 50 may not prove relatively worthy. There's no sunscreen that can give you all-day coverage. It doesn't exist. Also, an SPF of 50+ means the active ingredients are that much more concentrated, which makes the sunscreen potentially more likely to cause irritation, more side effects, and be harder to use.

- There is no such thing as a waterproof sunscreen, and the FDA finally regulated this erroneous claim. Sunscreens can only claim to be water-resistant now. This means you should reapply sunscreen after being in the water for more than fifteen minutes.

- As a cosmetic dermatologist in New York, and with 20 percent of my patients coming from abroad, I see all ethnicities. The most common après-sun complaint from those with darker skin is an uneven skin tone. My patients of color are often very surprised when I tell them to use sunscreen, as it will not only help protect them against skin cancer but will help prevent hyperpigmentation and

- blotchy areas. They might not need as *much* sunscreen as someone with fair skin, but they still need it!
- In addition to using mineral sunscreen, wearing a hat and/or protective clothing and staying in the shade are other safe forms of protection between the hours of 10:00 a.m. and 4:00 p.m.
- The best way to treat a sunburn is with aspirin or anti-inflammatories like Advil. In severe cases, topical cortisone creams or oral steroids will help. Moisturize with a basic cream. Don't pick at peeling skin. And vow to use more sunscreen next time you go to the beach!

Self-Tanners

When it's the dead of winter and my skin looks a bit green and pale under my office lights, I reach for the self-tanner. My patients are surprised when I recommend self-tanners, as they presume that all dermatologists would absolutely shun and shame any positive reinforcement we would give for having any hint of a tan. But self-tanners are actually safe when used topically, and quite effective. I think of them as a form of makeup—and a much better option than getting a tan.

The active ingredient in all self-tanners is DHA (dihydroxyacetone), a chemical compound that reacts with the amino acids in your topmost skin layer, the stratum corneum. It's basically just a topical dye of your dead-skin layer that sloughs itself off over time. (This is why it's always recommended to exfoliate before you apply a self-tanner, as this will get rid of the uneven layers of dead skin cells, so the lotion will be applied evenly. Areas that often get stained are the hands, knees, and elbows, where dead skin is thicker and harder to exfoliate. DHA is not physically absorbed, which is why it can be used after the first trimester of pregnancy. The formulations are constantly improving, so they're less orange, have less of an odor, and are mixed with antioxidants and other moisturizing ingredients to improve skin texture.

One of the complaints I frequently hear about self-tanners is that using them makes dark spots appear on the skin. That's because the spots were already there, due to sun damage, and the coloring of the self-tanner brings them out. (Obviously, if you notice a lot of spots, you should have a skin check by a dermatologist ASAP, just to be safe.) My solution is to get rid of patients' sun damage and resurface their skin, usually with a fractional laser. I had one patient in his seventies who was basically addicted to using a self-tanner, but his skin tone was so uneven and he had so many dark spots that he constantly switched products and then eventually baked in the sun. After convincing him to resurface his skin, after only two sessions he was cured of his unsuccessful habits. Now, the self-tanner gives him the skin tone he wants, and he doesn't have to go in the sun anymore to try to even it out.

There is one huge caveat with self-tanners that a lot of people don't know about. DHA is dangerous and carcinogenic if you inhale it. So if you go to a tanning booth, you *must* keep your mouth and nose covered and wear goggles. Especially if you're pregnant. (In fact, I tell women who are pregnant to never use spray tans, only topical lotion applied at home.) Always hold your breath when the spray is near your face.

The spraying should also be done in a well-ventilated area since the particles do stay in the air. Spray-tanning parlors are not filled with healthcare professionals or even licensed aestheticians who have to follow safety standards. There's no licensure program for spray tanning. Don't risk your life to get a fake tan!

How To Exercise Your Skin

Despite many claims to the contrary, you can't "exercise" your skin, because the muscles of your face, like the muscles of your gut, are different from those in your limbs. Striated muscles are the kind that you can exercise; they support bone structure and create lift when "built up" and strengthened, but they're not found in the face. The repetitive motion of facial exercises will just create wrinkles over time.

You *can*, however, do a slightly different form of exercise for your skin that doesn't give you the kind of workout you give your other muscles in the gym, but can still be effective. The right kind of exercise for your skin stimulates skin-cell turnover, builds collagen, and improves elasticity, which is why it's so effective.

There are many ways to get your skin "moving": physical or chemical exfoliation, manual devices such as rollers, and other devices that use light and heat.

Manual devices are deep-tissue massage devices and face and body rollers that you simply maneuver around the body. Using them improves lymphatic drainage and circulation, and doing so feels really good and relaxing as well. There are even home versions of LED lights that have no downtime and no side effects, but they are limited in their effects and best used as a follow-up to in-office visits, where the light and heat are stronger. We will see more of these home devices in the future.

For more advanced treatments that are performed in an office setting, you'll need to see a certified practitioner. These treatments create controlled damage of the skin and stimulate a repair mechanism; it's basically the same concept as strength training that breaks down muscle tissue so it can repair itself and become stronger. The best options are light and heat devices such as fractional resurfacing, intense pulsed light, radiofrequency, and ultrasound.

Pigmentation Issues: Lighteners and Brighteners

The biggest improvement you'll see with sun-induced hyper-pigmentation spots is what will happen when you start wearing sunscreen, especially on your face, neck, and hands. In the meantime, there have been amazing advances in lightening and brightening creams. There are prescription products that contain medicines such as hydroquinone and arbutin that, when used in moderation, can be effective and safe under the strict guidance of a dermatologist. Over-the-counter ingredients such as kojic acid, alpha and beta hydroxy acids, and newer ingredients such as tranexamic acid are very useful in helping to even out skin tone. Sadly, though, no cream is going to get rid of all your sunspots, only cosmetic procedures. You'll be waiting a whole lot longer than four to six weeks for that to happen if that is the expectation and desired result. Instead, go for a consultation with a dermatologist to see about removing the pigmentation by other means, especially if moderate or severe. Topical creams are certainly an excellent adjunct to treating various forms of hyperpigmentation by a dermatologist.

CHAPTER 2

Choosing Your Best Provider

Stay away from negative people.
They have a problem for every solution.

—ALBERT EINSTEIN

Rapid scientific developments and amazing advances in the last few years, for office treatments and over-the-counter products, means we can now use technology to mask the normal changes etched into skin by time in ways I never could have dreamed possible when I was in medical school.

As a result, the choices are great but there's too much redundancy. This is true whether you have skin cancer, wrinkles, or you're simply shopping for makeup. The average consumer doesn't have a medical education. They don't know what is effective and what is bogus. So much information floating around in the media is incorrect. Cosmetic surgery is the only field of medicine saturated with direct-to-consumer advertising in the media, so people come to me literally asking for a drug by name.

Because beauty is not just about procedures but about health and lifestyle, I tell all of my patients that they must be active participants in their consultation. My job is not to tell them what to do—it's to help them filter through the wide array of options.

In addition, I see the consultation as an opportunity to encourage all my patients to become part of the pro-aging community. I share expert advice that I want them to share with their families, friends, and colleagues. By educating and sharing, I increase the chances not only of giving great results to my patients, but also developing trust and long-lasting doctor/patient relationships.

Providers + Connection = A Must

Anyone considering any kind of treatment or procedure needs to be armed with as much information as possible before going to an appointment or consultation. Recommendations are always helpful, but how can you assess whether the practitioner is right for you? You always want the best one you can possibly find.

It starts with being a smart consumer. And, while I'm discussing the medical cosmetics arena specifically, the steps in this chapter should always be taken before you see *any* medical practitioner.

Remember: Cosmetic treatments are elective. You are in charge of choosing your provider, so take all the time you'll need to make informed choices. I want to emphasize that you *should* take your time and do due diligence. At least 10 percent of my practice is undoing botched procedures for very unhappy patients.

Even if you're not sure that cosmetic treatments are right for you at the moment, if you're contemplating some changes, a consultation with a qualified professional can be incredibly helpful, as you'll be given options that are appropriate for your age, lifestyle, health conditions, and budget. You will learn about treatments that you might not have read about. You might be told that what you actually need will cost far less than you expected. And, of course, you don't have to make immediate decisions.

You should never feel pressured, because the cosmetic arena is full of hype. I wish it weren't so, but there's a lot of false marketing for cosmetic procedures, and not everyone will have your best interests at heart. Anyone with a medical license can legally do cosmetic procedures, meaning dentists are doing injectables and gynecologists are doing hair and scar removal. Countless medical professionals—and, scarily enough, unlicensed and untrained quacks—want to get into the cosmetic game, for obvious reasons: cash-paying, healthy patients who just want to make themselves feel and look better.

The more you know, the less you'll spend and the less risk you'll have to deal with for treatments, procedures, and even over-the-counter products. The job of anyone you consult with is not just to tell you what the best is...because the best doesn't exist. Their job is to help you organize your treatment or your purchases in terms of priority in this order:

1. Safety
2. Best results
3. Best bang for your buck

Every Patient Is a Muse

How I reeducate my patients is very different to how cosmetic rejuvenation was practiced years ago. Then there were limited options: you went to the doctor, you listened, and that was it. This was true of all kinds of medicine. Now, with the technology and choices we have, my biggest goal is to teach you, learn about you, and help you develop your goals and prioritize the process.

This is a very important point for me, as developing a relationship with each person is what gets optimal results. The process starts *before* I put my gloves on. And it has nothing to do with how great a certain laser was for your friend or what you read about in *Vogue*. It has to do with trust, knowledge, and confidence that I'm giving you the best options for *you*. Because, after all, most cosmetic dermatologists may have the same toolbox of options, but they don't have the same skills at wielding them.

That's why, for me, every patient is a potential muse. They are generally interesting, accomplished people, whether they're traffic cops, teachers, job-seekers, retired moms and dads, celebrities, or masters of their financial universes. Having a doctor touch and manipulate their skin is intimate and brings us close together—literally and figuratively! They confide in me, and I harness my knowledge and skills to guide them. I am incredibly lucky to have such an amazing variety of patients in my life. They teach me as much as I teach them.

I hope that is the kind of relationship you will develop with your own practitioner. They should always want to see you again—and not because you're paying out of pocket. But because they know that *you* know how important self-care is.

Identify, Define, and Be Realistic About Your Needs

If you're not sure about what you want, or what's bothering you, how can you explain it to a dermatologist or any other kind of cosmetic healthcare provider?

While you're doing your due-diligence research about a cosmetic rejuvenation provider, it's time to have that conversation with yourself about what you are really looking for. Which ties into you being honest about your looks, your age, and your health.

Step One: Define Emotionally Whom *You're Doing It For*

My first question to new patients usually is, "Are you doing this for you, or are you doing it for someone else?" It's okay to want to look good for other people, but you also have to define what a treatment is going to do for *you*.

It's okay to want to look good for other people, but you also have to define what a treatment is going to do for you.

I have patients who've gone through a divorce, or have had health issues, or have lost or are changing jobs. They feel like they're seeing me for treatments because they "have to." My job is to empower them as to why they need to do this for themselves. Everything else comes along once you give yourself the power to acknowledge and believe in your own needs.

Some of the most satisfying treatments I do are with patients who come to me for the first time while recovering from physical or emotional challenges such as addiction or autoimmune disease and their health has now become stable, or after they've had chemotherapy to deal with their cancer. They're getting healthy again in remission, but they feel like they've been drained of everything and that their exterior doesn't match how they feel inside. They don't want to be seen as sick anymore, especially when they're on the mend.

These patients often feel bad, because they admit that they know they're lucky to be alive yet they somehow feel undeserving of a cosmetic or rejuvenating procedure. I tell them, "Listen, you've gone through a very internally brutal thing. Unfortunately, we still live in a world where we have to put poisons in our bodies to treat certain illnesses, but it's okay to try and fix the outside too, especially after going through such a brutal experience." We're visual creatures, and we don't want to be judged by someone who will treat us in a certain way if they think we're ill. Just as when, throughout much of the AIDS crisis, people suddenly became gaunt either from the illness itself or the medications used to treat it, and fillers were the best option to help them look better. The fillers removed the visual stigma and, at the time, the effects from the discrimination associated with AIDS.

Often, we can't stop ourselves from categorizing people and passing some sort of preconceived notion or judgment based on their external appearance; it's a human reflex. We have to teach people to be more accepting. There's nothing worse than knowing there's something wrong with somebody, and then not knowing what to say and looking away and making them feel more embarrassed.

Step Two: Define Emotionally Why You Want Something Done

I loved the TV show *Nip/Tuck* that was on the air from 2003 to 2010. It was a farcical drama about two plastic surgeons who weren't exactly role models for your ideal practitioner. Every episode opened with them saying to a patient, "Tell me what you don't like about yourself."

That always cracked me up—not exactly my technique! The first thing I do when I sit down at a new consultation is comment on a patient's *good* qualities. Only then can we focus on what bothers them, and then I can give them the best options.

A consultation is *not* just about what you see in the mirror—it's also about what's between your ears.

As you've read already, it's *not vanity* to want to look your best. It's *not vanity* to be unhappy with the visible signs of aging. Vanity is not synonymous with narcissism, it is merely the reward for self-care.

> *Vanity is not synonymous with narcissism, it is merely the reward for self-care.*

When it comes to your emotional needs, there are no wrong answers. For example, many men are less concerned with staying handsome or attractive; they're much more interested in staying competitive in the workforce, and they know that, as with women, ageism is a real problem. But they also want to stay competitive for their internal goals of remaining as vibrant and athletic-looking as possible.

Women, in my experience, feel deeply about body image, fear becoming less attractive, and are certainly pressured more by society to appear youthful. These feelings are intensely personal and can be hard to confront, even for the most accomplished and confident. This is neither fair nor deniable. This is where dealing with the emotions tied to cosmetic rejuvenation is essential in helping patients feel empowered rather than pressured.

Hopefully, clarifying your feelings about your appearance and the aging process will help you better manage all health-related issues as they arise, including aesthetic ones. That's what pro-aging is all about.

Step Three: Be as Honest and Realistic About Your Expectations as You Are About Your Needs

Wanting to look like somebody else, especially someone who's exceptionally gorgeous, is totally normal. Bringing a photograph of somebody else and asking for that face is not. There are limits to what cosmetic procedures can do. A little Botox at the tip of the nose can temporarily lift it, but I can't literally *reshape* your nose—only surgery can do that. Nor can I make a fifty-year-old look twenty-five again, but I can make her look like the best and most youthful version of herself at the age she is now.

Bringing in old photos is a good idea, as they'll show your practitioner what kind of youthful volume you once had in your face, and how much sun damage you might have—as long as you understand that these photos are a guideline, not a do-over!

Be realistic about expectations. Many practitioners do procedures that work, but if you get sold a procedure that, in the best-case scenario makes a 25 percent improvement on your wrinkles, yet you were expecting a 90 percent improvement, that discussion wasn't had. You're going to be unhappy. Expectations and results can vary tremendously. Not just on the treatment, but also due to your age, your skin type, your anatomy, and any underlying health issues.

Set realistic goals in your mind *before* you see your practitioner, and you're much less likely to be disappointed.

When Is the Right Time to Seek Cosmetic Treatments?

When someone asks me, "When do I start?" I always say: "You start when things start to bother you."

The level of *bother*, of course, is something only you can answer.

Pro-aging means you become the best version of *you*, at any age. It's easy to be twenty years old. When I discuss issues with a millennial, my focus is about how they're in it for the long haul; they have their lives ahead of them. Treatments should be preventative. The smart millennials are going to say, "Is this going to affect the way I look when I'm fifty?"

And then I tell them, "Not the way I do it!" The majority come to me for body treatments, as they usually aren't unhappy with their faces yet—which I find very ironic because they'll spend the rest of their lives wishing they have the body they had right then.

> *When someone asks me, "When do I start?" I always say:*
> *"You start when things start to bother you." The level of*
> *bother, of course, is something only you can answer.*

As people get older, they get more concerned about their faces. That usually starts when they're in their late twenties, thirties, or early forties. When I speak to someone in their fifties and beyond, it's usually about how to get them back to ten years ago.

When I discuss subtle but significant changes, a lot of my new patients still fret that someone will "notice" that they've had a procedure. That's one of the biggest reasons why people elect *not* to have any treatments. First off, you only are noticing the *bad work* out there. Second, *you* are the only person who matters anyway. If people look overdone or fake, it's usually not because of how much they had done—it's because of how much *of one thing* they had done. One patient might get just one syringe of filler in one cheek and look like a cosmetic-surgery victim. Another patient might get ten syringes, but, if put in many different places, they'll still look like themselves, only better. If I just paint one wall bright white, every other wall is going to look dirty, no matter how clean it is. That's what people notice: something that stands out. You have to look at life like that. Put a little paint on every wall to have an overall striking result.

It's never too late to seek advice either. Obviously, the older you are, the more extensive your treatment plan might be. Or not. Some of the most beautiful and content people I know have never had a professional do anything to their faces.

Many patients ask, "How much is enough?" I always tell them that as long as they're not distorting themselves, it makes them feel good about themselves, and it impacts their sense of well-being in a positive way, then don't worry about doing too much. Just go to a professional with the judgment, skill, and respect for their needs to put the brakes on things when need be.

As for knowing if you should stop doing things altogether at some point, unfortunately, at any stage of life, "letting yourself go" is usually a result of intense stress or illness. Because of this, we must recognize that, at any age, the ability to groom ourselves and to care for our appearance is always a blessing. Beauty and health always shine from within. As humans, we reflexively strive for our reflection to match.

Write It Down

If you find it hard to talk about deeply personal issues of body image and fears, it often helps to write out a list first, rewrite it as much as needed, then bring the list to the appointment with you, so you can refer to your notes. Going to see someone to discuss elective procedures can be very stressful. In moments like these, it's very easy to forget some or all of your questions.

I actually like it when patients pull out a list. It means they've been doing their homework, and that makes the consultation more efficient and effective.

This is a good habit to get into whenever you go to see any kind of medical practitioner.

It's okay to ask a doctor questions such as: "How many times a day do you do this procedure?" and "How many years have you been doing this procedure?" No doctor should balk at these questions. Especially if you're going to someone that you have not found by word of mouth.

I also love patients who are direct about their needs and are open to me educating them about the possibilities. They might not like what I have to say sometimes—which is often no, if they ask for something unrealistic or that won't help them!—but at least we can have an honest and productive conversation about what might work instead.

No matter what your budget is, I want you to guide me, so I can get to know you and your goals better to give you the best possible treatment.

How to Find a Cosmetic Healthcare Provider

My job is not just education, as you know, but *reeducation*. Why? Because the beauty business is booming. It's the Wild West out there. It's confusing for patients, and it's often confusing for doctors. Every state has different regulations about who can do what, and where, and I've realized that even a lot of doctors aren't up to date about these laws. So before you set foot in any practitioner's office, a little bit of homework is a must.

The Pre-Appointment Checklist

Specialty Training and Licensure Are Crucial

Just because any licensed MD can legally perform cosmetic procedures doesn't mean you want your gynecologist wielding a laser to tighten up your creepy neck!

Basic Medical Training for the Doctor

Experts in aesthetic treatments have to be thoroughly trained and experienced in the actual health of whatever they're doing. Cosmetic dermatologists go through general internal medicine and general dermatology first. Plastic surgeons go through general surgical training first. You cannot be a safe or quality cosmetic provider unless you know and understand the health ramifications of procedures and the various medical diseases and treatments of the skin. I always say to my patients, "It's easy when everything goes right. The skill of a healthcare provider is often revealed when things go wrong. And in any form of medicine, things do go wrong occasionally."

Aesthetic healthcare is an extra level of training above and beyond the basic levels of dermatology and plastic surgery, ophthalmology, or ENT. The cosmetic provider you choose should have had general training in one these specialties, followed by extra fellowships or training in cosmetic, aesthetic treatments.

This is often misconstrued because there are aesthetic providers out there who don't go through the extra training. There are a lot of other specialties, such as OB/GYN, ER, internal medicine, or various other family practices, that are noncore specialties, and these doctors are trying to learn aesthetic procedures purely for financial gain. They take a course or two and suddenly think they're qualified to be aesthetic doctors.

Basic Medical Training for the Staff

It's very important to ask where the provider's staff was trained. If you are seeking care from a nurse practitioner, a registered nurse, or a physician assistant (PA)—the nonphysician providers for aesthetic healthcare—you need to know that they not only have training and experience in aesthetic medicine, but they have had thorough experience in the core general specialties and understand the medical health and treatment of the skin. Qualified practitioners have worked with plastic surgeons or dermatologists for years prior to cosmetic training and performance. For me, five to ten years is a minimum of prior experience in both the core specialty and aesthetic healthcare.

Research Certification and Licensure

After doctors graduate from medical school, they must first pass board examinations in order to get their medical license. You'll want to know when the license was issued and what additional certifications, such as a board certification in various specialties— which means years of additional training in a teaching hospital. I am always happy to share that I spent four years in medical school, followed by one year of internal medicine and three years in dermatology training, and then one year of advanced cosmetic training with my mentor. Followed by eighteen years of private practice and teaching professorships at major resident teaching hospitals.

One of the best resources with information about who can treat, for consumers and for doctors, is the American Med Spa Association (AMSPA) at americanmedspa.org. They are doing the best they can to tame the confusion by creating a resource, as well as lobbying politically to help standardize state laws to provide oversight and ensure physicians are doing what they're supposed to be doing. The Resources tab is extremely helpful.

Research the Specialties

Look for specialty training, as well as how long this practitioner has been doing the procedures you're interested in. Is their training in plastic surgery or cosmetic dermatology? Is their expertise with filler or lasers? Do they do only facial procedures or whole-body? You don't want to go to someone who touts themselves as a jack-of-all-trades, as they're more likely to be a master of none.

Find Out Who Actually Does the Procedures

Websites should list the credentials of all the employees performing the procedures, as well as list the site's licensed MD who has been involved in the training and oversight of the practice. If not, pick up the phone and ask!

I can't stress how crucial this is.

There are med spas and storefronts offering aesthetic treatments that can be lifesavers or face-wreckers. They are more likely to be face-wreckers if there's no ready accessibility to a board-certified physician. This physician doesn't have to be the one performing the procedure, but there has to be a clear signage and availability of a physician if need be, at all times.

There are med spas all over the country that do not list any of that. If so, they are breaking the law. You can't do PR or marketing for any type of medical procedure without the credentials and visibility of a licensed doctor. Never ever go to any practice that doesn't provide this very basic information. *All forms of cosmetic enhancement are the practice of medicine.* Don't be fooled by nice couches and pretty flowers and gushing testimonials.

In other words, no matter how much it looks like a fancy salon, a med spa, or any other kind of business offering injectables, lasers, or non-superficial peels, it should still be a doctor's office. Not only by ethics but by *law*. And even though there doesn't have to be a doctor on-site 24/7, there must be a medical director, and the responsibility always lies on that doctor. At any point in time, you should have access to that doctor. You always have to have your questions answered, and if they're not answered by a licensed healthcare practitioner, they must be by a physician that's overseeing the treatment. If you walk in to a laser place in New York State, you have to have access to a physician, if you want, and you have to be evaluated.

You always have that right, but very few consumers know this. This regulation is not enforced, in large part because laws vary by state. For example, in New York State a nurse can do any of the procedures that I do, but not without a doctor seeing the patient first and going through a health history and what the procedure entails. These nurses may be as skilled as a doctor, but the doctor *must* give the okay to the nurse before your treatment. Except for laser hair removal, which New York State doesn't consider a medical procedure, so anyone with training can do it. But in New Jersey, all laser treatments are considered medical procedures, and only a doctor can perform them.

Because there's very poor regulation, people assume that if they go to a place that has a nice website and environment, all the provider's credentials will be in order and there won't be any risk. There are a lot of nonphysicians performing procedures without a doctor on site. That is illegal.

Understand Licensing Terminology and Who Can Legally Do What in Your State

There is also a lot of confusion about licenses and terminology. There are two types:

- *A licensed esthetician,* who is trained in a vocational specific school.
- *A licensed medical healthcare provider.* This includes doctors, nurses, nurse practitioners, and PAs.

There is no license for a "medical aesthetician." That term is a scam.

I love aestheticians. They're highly skilled and provide an amazing complement to the things I do. Unfortunately, however, aestheticians are trying to expand their cosmetic game because they're worried about becoming obsolete. Many take laser courses and get certificates and tell people they are licensed and trained to do these procedures in their state when they actually are not. A certificate from a laser company is not a license to perform that procedure. A license makes the bearer legally responsible for any problems and holds them to a certain standard. However, many of these aestheticians work for med spas run by financial investors and have no doctor present. They get sued, they go bankrupt, they run...and you have no legal recourse.

In some states, aestheticians and medical assistants can perform laser procedures; I think this is nutty and dangerous.

If a technology or a drug is serious enough to be recognized and regulated by the FDA, then I believe it should require the licensure of a healthcare professional to perform the treatment. During the FDA approval process, it's doctors, nurses, and PAs that are doing the trials. Not aestheticians and other non-healthcare assistants.

Bear in mind that FDA approval doesn't mean a treatment *works*. FDA approval means only that it's been deemed relatively safe for consumer treatment. It's a *safety* issue—not an *effectiveness* issue.

My medical assistants and aestheticians are an integral, complimentary part of the medical care provided in my office. But they're not healthcare professionals upheld by the licensure and training recognized by the State of New York. Physicians, nurses, registered nurses, physician assistants, and nurse practitioners are.

The Difference Between Aesthetic Treatments and Medical Treatments

In my opinion, all aesthetic treatments that require consent and have risks and benefits must be performed by a licensed healthcare provider. Any treatment that goes significantly below the epidermis, the superficial top layer of the skin, and has a biological effect on the deeper, living layers of the skin, is a medical procedure and carries medical risks and benefits. That's how it's defined in most states, and regardless of what is loosely allowed or loopholed in some states, that is how I define it after my decades of practice and seeing the full spectrum of the good, the bad, the risks, and the complications.

So if you're considering going to anyone other than a licensed MD for your treatments, look for this information:

- Who the medical director is. If no one is listed, run.
- If there is only a bare-bones website that doesn't provide thorough information about the medical oversight, run.
- The training and support of the medical staff. If you go somewhere that doesn't have a staff of licensed healthcare professionals to perform the treatments, run. If they don't want to share that information with you, run. They are breaking the law.

- If they have only one device or one or two treatments, or if they don't talk about customized treatments overseen by a licensed, experienced physician, run.

A med spa is just a different name for a doctor's office. Any med spa that tries to de-emphasize the nature of the medical treatment and the support that's required is not a med spa for you. Legally, physically, and ethically. Quality and safety are the most important factors. The face you save may be your own!

There are many good providers out there. Consumers should be given safe options other than traditional doctor's offices. The cosmetic market is changing and growing rapidly, and the audience is growing and diversifying. My vision is to create legitimate sources of care for the full range of consumers, places where the best technology, medical oversight, customized treatments, and quality of care is given by licensed healthcare providers at a reasonable cost. Hopefully, this is where the future of beauty lies.

Check Out Websites and Digital Media

Look for Details on the Practitioner's Website

Google the doctor's website for basic information, but realize that a high-quality website doesn't mean the doctor is high quality. Always look for the doctor's professional training, board certification, licensure, and membership in professional organizations.

Assessing Before and After Photos

It's very informative to look through these photos to see the very visible changes after treatments. I use them to help explain certain procedures and show my patients the type of result they can get, but I don't use them solely as a sales tool for new patients. Because these images can also be easily altered now in ways that were much more difficult to do even a few years ago. In addition, doctors are always going to show you the top 1 percent of their patients with the top results. You're never going to see anything botched or ineptly done.

So when you're assessing before and after photos, make sure the patient is in the exact same position, with the exact same facial expression. The lighting should be the same. The patient should have no makeup or jewelry on. Hair should be pulled away from the face. You can't judge somebody if they're frowning in the before photo but smiling in the after photo, or if they have no makeup on in the before shot and lots of it on in the after.

Be Skeptical of Consumer-Driven Websites and Media

You can obtain valuable information from sites like Yelp and RealSelf, but you have to realize that it can be highly biased. As you likely know from Yelp's restaurant reviews, opinions are highly personal and often inaccurate. Especially if the reviewer had unrealistic expectations.

The same goes for magazines or websites with beauty coverage. They are funded primarily by ad revenue, and they are not going to bite the hands that feed them with controversial or unflattering stories about their advertisers' products or procedures. Media outlets have a different agenda when touting the newest technology or treatment. Most important for them is to be the first to mention something. They are far less concerned with whether or not the trendiest new thing actually works over the long term.

Be Even More Skeptical about Social Media

Unfortunately, we live in a world of social media and fancy websites. No way should you judge a book totally by its cover, especially when it seems that everyone's got a fabulous life on Instagram. We don't, of course, know the demons inside, or whether the photos and stories were staged, Photoshopped, or entirely fictitious. You have to be wary because we're thrown so much glossy content, and social media is driven by clicks and followers (who can, of course, be fake). The people you follow can be incredibly helpful and informative (which is what I hope my Instagram feed is!), but you have to look at many other sites or feeds with a healthy dose of skepticism. They're not always to be taken at face value; they can create a façade of legitimacy that doesn't exist in real life.

Be very cautious of anything that looks too good or too bad to be true. It's way too easy to manipulate and add filters to images now.

Be the Most Skeptical about Deeply Discounted or Groupon Skincare "Specials"

Those special offers certainly sound amazing. But whoever's selling the Groupon treatment is doing it at cost to get patients in, so they can sell them other, more profitable treatments, or just plain practice on them. No person with experience or expertise is going to do a Groupon because they won't make a penny. Injectables, lasers, and other cosmetic devices cost money. They are not a cheap addition to the doctors' overhead. So if a treatment sounds too cheap to be true—guess what—it is.

When other doctors ask my advice about marketing and coupons, I tell them that the type of person who will come in from Groupon is a one-time customer. They're not going to say, "Oh, you did such a good job I'll pay a lot more next time." No, they're going to go to the next Groupon. This is probably the biggest no-no I can share about finding a cosmetic provider. It doesn't serve the doctor or the patient well at all.

Word of Mouth

It's always great to seek the advice of friends, especially if they look wonderful after the treatments they had and were happy with their care. They can also give you a realistic assessment of the provider's bedside manner, the treatments offered, the office environment, and the staff.

And, as I'll discuss at length later in this chapter, you have to realize that your friend's treatments may not have the same type of result or impact on you because everyone's skin and health are different. There are limitations based on anatomy, age, the type of wrinkles, sun exposure, and skin tone. I can't get the exact same results on two best friends of the same age. Or even on identical twins!

Everyone's response is different. Use word of mouth for what it's worth, and then realize you have to take your own journey—one you'll want to develop with your practitioner.

Also, sometimes there are kickbacks paid either directly or in the form of free treatments—an illegal but common practice—for word-of-mouth recommendations, which is something you likely will never know.

Now don't get me wrong. All these above facts are true, but as many of you know, I clearly participate in social media, marketing, and publicity. I try my best to educate rather than exaggerate, and sometimes I wish people spent more time looking at my walls of diplomas than they do my social media! Clearly, it's all pieces of a puzzle. Schooling and training, years of experience, word of mouth, and *quality* of experience are still the most important criteria. Ultimately, it's about feeling comfortable and well cared-for. In the end, it still is the practice of medicine. Do your research as if your health depended on it...because it does!

> *Ultimately, it's about feeling comfortable and well cared-for.*

The Price Is Not Always Right

Don't make decisions about any procedures, treatments, or products based *purely* on price. There are many factors which go into pricing—the cost of the drugs and devices, location, and experience, for example. A newly minted dermatologist who's just starting to build a practice could have a high skill level but cost far less than the highly touted, much older physician with a great PR team and lousy results.

Few websites list prices because they can change so often, but if you call a doctor's office, you should be given an approximate price range. I wouldn't recommend that you go anywhere where you're quoted a definitive figure, as there's no way of assessing what you really need until you're having an in-person consultation. Bait and switch is not uncommon either, especially if you just want a filler and are given a good price just to get you in the door, and then the price has somehow changed overnight.

In the beauty business, you don't always get what you pay for. You know this if you've shopped for a new moisturizer and found prices ranging from a few dollars up to a thousand for a small jar of cream. Does a cream that costs fifty times another work fifty times better? Not quite.

But you also need to know that pharmaceutical drugs and devices do cost a significant amount of money to the provider. (Lasers can cost several hundred thousand dollars, for instance.) If, however, you see anything that's significantly lower within the price spectrum, there's a reason for it: it's diluted or illegal. There are non-FDA-approved products and devices being imported from China and elsewhere all the time. I know of clinics near my office that are injecting artificial Botox and fillers they bought off the internet. It's *dangerous*! But they wouldn't be doing it if they didn't have customers willing to pay less—and unwittingly get less.

Do you want an illegal, diluted drug injected into your face? I don't think so!

In The Cosmetic Healthcare Provider's Office

Once you've done your due diligence for the pre-appointment checklist, it's time to move on to the actual appointment. Cosmetic procedures are elective. You are in charge of finding a practitioner who is not only skilled, but makes you feel good during the entire process, because you're paying out of pocket for it. If there are any red flags, say goodbye and find someone else!

The Office Environment Is Important

You have to feel safe and welcome. That's part of the whole office demeanor. If you walk in to see beautiful flowers and the waiting room is comfortable and smells good, that's great. It will help you relax and make you feel valued, as you should feel!

The bathroom and the entire office should be spotless. No matter how lovely the décor, you are still in a doctor's office, and hygiene is paramount.

The Staff's Attitude Is Important

You should always be treated with kindness and respect. Rude or unhelpful staff is a huge red flag. If the staff treats you this way, what does it say about their boss?

One big problem is lateness. This is a huge problem for all doctors and surgeons; if the early appointments show up late, there can be a cascade effect of backing up the rest of the day. And one emergency can throw things off completely. How the staff manages you needing to wait is another indication of the provider's quality of care.

Your Privacy Is Super Important

Not long ago, a new med spa opened downtown, with only a curtain between the treatment rooms. I couldn't believe it. What if a woman was talking about her private health history? What if a patient was expressing pain or bleeding?

A curtain is not an option. There are federal HIPAA (Health Insurance Portability and Accountability Act) laws regarding your privacy for a reason. There *must* be privacy between the treatment rooms, so you can be assured of doctor/patient confidentiality. You should not be able to hear conversations in any other room or hallway. There must be closed doors. Your chart should never be faceup on the outside of the door to the treatment room so other people can see your name. This is for your protection.

Give any practitioner who's cavalier about your privacy the boot!

Your Practitioner Should Always Know More than You Think You Do—So Please Don't Self-Diagnose!

The ideal patient is one who walks into my office with their list. It shows me they've done their homework, have realistic expectations, and want informed answers about informed questions. They become an active participant, not just in the initial consultation, but for all ensuing treatments.

On the other hand, some patients trip themselves up. On *their* list: wanting the same procedures their friends had done. They bring in copies of articles or pictures of celebrities touting the latest, trendiest treatments; information they've gotten from watching YouTube and Instagram; names of specific treatments and specific devices; even names of specific drugs.

If you have cancer, can you imagine going to your oncologist and demanding Taxol or Cytoxan for your chemotherapy? Of course you wouldn't. A person with cancer goes to an oncologist who evaluates all the variables and the type/stage of disease, and then draws upon their training and experience to deliver the treatment they think best. It is great to become educated about all your options and do your own research, but you have to stay open-minded.

It should be like that with cosmetic rejuvenation too. A good practitioner will tell you there's not just one answer to any problem. It's more important for you to say, "This is what bothers me," instead of, "I really need Fraxel because my BFF just had it with Doctor So-and-So, and she looks really great."

Be smart about what you can be smart about. That's *your* job. You're buying a professional's judgment and experience and, hopefully, the results you seek. You're not buying a device or a dose of a particular drug you read about in a magazine.

Often, patients ask, "Dr. Frank, do you have this laser I saw online?" If I say no, they'll say, "Well, should I go to my friend's doctor who has this laser and have my face done there?"

I tell them that aesthetic medicine is 100 percent of my practice. I already have thirty-five different devices in my office. I try all the new devices. If I think it's going to make cosmetic improvement, be safe, and help grow my practice, well, of course, I'm buying that device. I choose my artillery based on my belief in it. If I don't buy it, I don't believe in it. A device may work for someone else's practice, but my job and my own business is to find things that are not only going to make money, but that I believe in because I have the proof that they really work and offer a realistic and safe option for my patients.

For example, a lot of people come in for skin tightening, not wanting fillers, which require maintenance, and I have to convince them fillers would be better, especially if their faces are hollowed. I tell them I'm not going to charge $5,000 for something that's going to make a 10 percent difference. I'd rather see them spend half the amount and make a significant difference because their problem is volume, not loose skin. Or some patients come in for filler, but they have very round faces, so they need more skin tightening. The good news with skin tightening is, although it's more expensive, there's less maintenance involved.

That's where misinformation comes in. There is no "one size fits all." I'm trying to be cost-effective and give patients a happier result because I don't want them to be unsatisfied. The point is, these patients sometimes erroneously self-diagnosed, and it's up to me to explain why. Hopefully, my expertise will save them time, money, and pain and give them the results they seek. When they follow my advice and decide to have a procedure I tell them is best for them, it's because I want to find the safest, most effective, and most cost-effective way to reach our end goal. They don't know the technology that I know about. Sometimes, they do need the more expensive, riskier, more downtime treatment. Sometimes they need much less.

We live in a very direct-to-consumer cosmetic market. We see ads for Botox and Fraxel and countless other drugs and treatments. We are bombarded with articles and postings. But whenever you decide to make cosmetic treatments a part of your pro-aging protocol, you're buying a *service*. It's not necessarily the brand of paint or the instrument, it's the artist that gives the end result. You want good quality, but you have to let the doctor choose the shades and thicknesses of their "paint" and play you the song *they* choose.

Remember: Drugs used for cosmetic dermatology are still drugs. The treatments might be elective and sound benign, but as I've said many times already, they are still medical procedures. People don't think of cosmetic treatments like they do general medicine. Your doctor or practitioner should always know far, *far* more than you ever will.

You Must Be Given Options, Because the Best Treatment/Procedure Is the One that Works for You

It's incredibly gratifying that we live in a world today where there are so many pro-aging options, whether in my office or that you can do at home. But just because a procedure exists doesn't mean it works...and, even if it does work, it doesn't mean it will work for you. Remember: in the end, you're not buying a result, but options, judgment, expertise, and a service.

This conversation is one I have with my patients every single day. If I have a hundred patients with the same complaint, they're all going to benefit from different kinds of treatments because there's no single solution to any beauty or wellness need. If you only have a hammer, everything looks like a nail...so make sure you go to someone with a full tool chest. You can't go to a doctor who only has one trick or who has one laser and says it can do everything. There's no such thing. A jack-of-all-trades is often a master of none.

> *If you only have a hammer, everything looks like a nail...*
> *so make sure you go to someone with a full tool chest.*

When You Hear No, Be Happy and Say Yes

"No" is a word I often say to my patients.

I say no to Botox if you don't have wrinkles. I often say no to laser if you don't have sun damage. It's fantastic that my patients are getting younger and thinking about pro-aging prophylactically, but that doesn't mean they need what they think they might.

Sometimes, patients are happy and confident with what I've already done, but they still want more. For them, a point arrives where I have to refuse to do what they ask. I know the treatment in question will either not be needed; it will end up looking fake;

they will get better results if, perhaps, I try something else in a different area; or they need to consult a plastic surgeon for a more invasive procedure. Or they might need to deal with psychological issues about their appearance if they start having unrealistic expectations or are overly concerned about their appearance.

Sometimes these patients listen to me. Sometimes they don't. They can always find another practitioner who will give them what they want. If they do this and come back to me, I won't treat them. A patient who won't listen to my advice is a patient who will never be satisfied, and that's not good for either of us.

Think About the Long Term

I've been practicing long enough to know that short-term results are not the only results to consider. Everything has short- and long-term consequences. Don't let anyone tell you that immediate gratification is all that matters. It isn't!

There are many long-term factors to consider. How does this person age? Family genetics will always come into play. What if this person wants a facelift in the future? What is this person's stress level? What technological developments might be on the horizon? How long has this hot new laser been around? Do we know if there might be long-term repercussions to its use? What about this drug? How long had it been tested before being FDA-approved?

Medicine can be a miraculous lifesaver, but it is not infallible. The FDA sometimes approves drugs or devices that are later withdrawn due to damaging side effects. Certain types of permanent breast or wrinkle implants have proven harmful and subsequently have been recalled, for example, yet no one thought there'd be an issue when they first went into use. When Prozac was released twenty years ago, mental health professionals thought it was the biggest wonder drug in the world, but now they've realized that its long-term side effects and efficacy are similar to older anti-depressants. Or might not even be as good. Do I even have to mention the story of OxyContin—the supposed wonder drug for pain relief that has led to the biggest opioid crisis this country has ever seen?

Everything has long-term consequences, and it's up to you to have a candid discussion about the risks and checks and balances with your practitioner. You need to get honest answers. Better to err on the safe side than to be a guinea pig for something you'll soon regret.

Never, Ever Have Any Procedures Done Outside of a Medical Office

Before the internet was invented, people often said New York was the city that never sleeps. That's still true, but the internet is always open too. Not only can you order things you want 24/7, but you can order things you never should. I know of people who have ordered medical-grade chemical peels (unavailable OTC as they are prescription-only) online, watched a YouTube how-to video, did the peel at home, and ended up burned, scarred, and permanently disfigured.

I have no doubt that the procedures I do easily give my patients the results they seek, but they are still never 100 percent safe or without a chance of side effects or bad results. They require expertise and, always, a high level of caution.

About 10 percent of my practice is seeing complications. Eight times out of ten, it's because the patient said, "My friends went to go see this person. I thought they had a good experience. I had no idea this person legally couldn't do these shots or use that laser. I didn't know they weren't a doctor or some trained person."

Be wary. Medical procedures should never be done outside of a controlled medical environment. *Never.* Not in luxury homes, not in apartments, not in hotel rooms. Some people have invite-only Botox parties, which can be a safety issue.

Sometimes the person doing the injecting isn't even a doctor. Your home or hotel is hardly a sterile environment. Your privacy will be exposed. People can lie about their health conditions and prior treatments, which can cause problems. If there are complications, you could have serious consequences without the appropriate treatment measures available. The issue isn't when things go right, but when things go wrong. Then what do you do? If you're in a medical environment, the staff should be trained to handle any complication or emergency, such as fainting, allergic reactions, or worse.

There are countless stories about Botox parties at someone's house where there was drinking. That's crazy! Alcohol makes you bruise more easily. It affects your judgment. Consenting to get any treatment is a judgment. You have to be lucid when this conversation is taking place.

Be smart. Be safe!

New Isn't Necessarily Better

As you've learned already, people read or hear about a new filler or a new laser, and they ask me why I haven't told them about these trendy things. I tell them I *do* have that filler and that laser, but I'd only tell them about it if I thought it would be good for them—because what we've been using for the last four years works *better*.

If it ain't broke, don't fix it; and new is not always better—that new thing could end up harming you. Which is why I tell those who are susceptible to social pressures and over-hyped fads, "Check yourself before you wreck yourself!"

Hype about newness can be particularly dangerous with medical procedures. The hottest technique may not have been around long enough to determine its safety and efficacy. Just because it's approved by the FDA doesn't mean that it works or works over time. Data on regular use and effectiveness can only be compiled after several years of use.

After practicing for twenty years, I like to remain on the cutting edge and have new things, but as much as I love new technology, I'm always wary of it until long-term results are in. Ultimately, I have to do my own research. You want to go to a provider who does the same, and still has the tried-and-true as an option.

New fillers come out all the time. That doesn't mean they're better. When I was doing my residency, Gore-Tex lip implants were the hot thing. But they turned out to be horrible. They became hard, they shifted position, they looked fake. People who'd gotten them needed surgery to have them removed.

For example, new Botox-like neuromodulators have been coming out, such as Jeuveau, Xeomin, and Dysport, and, of course, I use them where appropriate. But I only change things up on patients who no longer get the same results that they used to with the other available neuromodulators. Or, if I decide to get a new laser, I won't offer it to the Fraxel patient who's been coming to me once a year for the past five years and loves the results. The patient that I may try a new laser on is someone who may not have responded to prior treatments with earlier technologies. That's where new may be better.

Stick with the basics. New devices, in particular, are extremely expensive. A doctor who's just bought a trendy new $100,000 laser is going to want to pay it off. Just realize that many treatments, drugs, and lasers come and go, just as many businesses in other fields seem initially successful but close up shop if they don't stand the test of time.

Noninvasive Is Not Always Best Either

Many people have a preconceived idea that noninvasive procedures are always better and less risky than invasive procedures, such as surgery. Trust me on this: They're not. Or, rather, they are sometimes.

You can you spend a lot more time and trauma healing and get less-than-stellar results with a noninvasive procedure. I do a lot of neck liposuction, for instance, under local anesthesia. In an hour, I can remove 90 percent of the fat, and the patient can go back to work two days later. I hate to tell this to patients who come to me after they've endured five $2,000 treatments of Kybella, an injectable treatment to dissolve fat under the chin. It can work—but never as well as liposuction—and it can also leave patients extremely swollen for over a week after each of the five injections. Whereas I could make one little incision and, an hour later, it's all over!

There are also skin-tightening procedures I do for forty-year-olds that work wonderfully well. But then a seventy-year-old patient will come in and tell me that her doctor charged her thousands of dollars to do the same treatment that not only didn't work but was extremely painful. She felt scammed. What she needed was a facelift. If she hadn't wanted a facelift, fair enough. She should never have been sold a treatment that her doctor knew was inappropriate.

If you're at an age or have severe issues which don't have a lot of noninvasive options that will work effectively to treat them, invasive surgery may be the only option for optimal results. At that point, you need to discuss all your options with your doctor. It's totally understandable to not want surgery. Fortunately, new advances in treatments and devices are being released all the time. I can do things now that I couldn't do a mere five years ago! The perfect treatment for you might be out there before you know it.

Informed Consent Is a Must

Never get sold any treatment unless you are asked for informed consent. This is a must for *every* medical procedure.

A consent form explains the risks involved in the procedure you're choosing. You need to know about them, in case something goes wrong. The forms can be scary, and people get anxious reading them, because they deal with the worst-case scenarios of even very simple procedures. Still, you need to be told about the realistic risks and benefits and not have them blown off as impossibilities. Which is why it's not only illegal but also incredibly stupid for any practitioner to not provide informed consent.

Most severe complications that you'll see on the consent form about the procedures I do are extremely rare. But if the complication happened one time to one patient somewhere in the world, it has to be listed on the form. Most of the common complications are less severe and for the most part manageable by skilled practitioners.

Some people don't bother to read the forms and sign them with a shrug. Others read them and say, in a panic-stricken voice, "Fillers can make me blind?" Yes, they can, if they get trapped inside a blood vessel and block the blood supply to your optic nerve. Yes, there are such cases in the literature, but I've never seen one. I can tell you with confidence that I've injected filler into every adult member of my family, including myself, and that I think the cost-to-benefit ratio of doing so makes it a very safe procedure relative to other forms of surgical intervention, let alone just walking down the street. In fact, I believe for all intents and purposes that there's a greater chance of being struck by lightning then there is of going blind from filler injected by the right provider.

Regardless, read the consent form, ask questions, and have the discussion.

If You Get a Hard Sell, Run!

Any good healthcare provider, makeup counter person, skincare expert, or aesthetician will first get an idea during the consultation of what your needs are before they recommend anything. You need to be given options, not just a sales pitch.

The hard sell is one of the biggest red flags to watch for. Be wary. This is not retail. If someone is overselling you, they are not working in your best interest.

You must be offered multiple options for any issue you have. Anyone who tells you that only "this" device or product will work, or that you need to schedule treatment "right away," is a problem. That might be true of medical conditions, like a cancerous mole, but not for elective cosmetic procedures.

Good doctors have busy practices. They don't need to hard-sell any of their services. There are abuses in my line of work; it's my job to prevent people from going overboard. That is the responsibility of all practitioners who choose to give this kind of care. I take and own that responsibility for my patients and for myself.

Don't Lie

Just as hard-sell practitioners lie about treatments, patients also can lie. So many of my new patients used to lie about their age that I now ask for a driver's license before I see anyone. I totally understand someone wanting to fudge their age; we live in an ageist society where judgments about age are swift. But not in a medical office.

Lying can cause you grave harm. People lie about chronic illnesses. People lie about how much they drink or take drugs. People lie about the prescription medications they take, which can be contraindicated to something I might prescribe. People lie about previous work they've had done—even when I can see the scars! That makes it hard for me to have an honest relationship with someone and provide my best judgment.

Don't Go to Different Providers for the Same Treatment

It's not a good idea to have similar treatments done by different providers. If you like and trust one particular provider, let them be the only chef in the kitchen—otherwise, it makes it difficult for that provider to give you their best work. You want treatments that are customized to you, whether you're going to a great aesthetician, nutritionist, fitness coach, or cosmetic dermatologist. One size doesn't fit all, so how can you expect customized care if you have different people performing it? It's like going to a different tailor who measures you differently for your suits. Nothing will fit the same way.

You can't change the members of the band every time you play the band's song, but there will always be some people who keep looking for a better deal and are switching it up. When they come back to see me, I won't treat them anymore because I won't tolerate patients who lie about it. It's not about ego at all. It's because every practitioner has their own technique, dosing, and aesthetic. If a patient has a complication, I won't know what's in their face if someone else did their treatments! Consistency with the same providers is important.

Discussing the Pain Factor

Pain is a 100 percent subjective phenomenon.

Significant pain is the biggest signal that something is not going well. Nothing that a cosmetic healthcare provider does should ever be intolerably painful. If it is, then it's the fault of the doctor. I've had patients who come in and tell me they're afraid of certain lasers because their friends got treated and said the pain was terrible. Pain control is essential to any procedure. I believe it when people are screaming in pain, and I believe it when people say they don't feel a thing—so for first-time patients, I use as many pain-modifying techniques as possible. Options are topical anesthesia, mild forms of sedation, distraction tools, skin-cooling devices, and laughing gas, among other forms of distraction.

If you're worried, speak up! It's totally normal to be anxious about something that might be painful. My goal is always to make the biggest scaredy-cats into the most comfortable patients, especially for needle-phobics. Some people freeze at the mere sight of a syringe. Techniques from simple "talkesthesia" all the way to drug-induced sedation are options to get people comfortably through any procedure. A comfortable patient allows a skilled provider to do their best work. Discomfort and squirming help no one and can actually increase the risk of bruising and poor cosmetic outcomes.

There is also a lot of psychology behind what hurts and what doesn't. Some patients have multiple injections, several laser sessions, and lots of other treatments that can sting a little, and they don't even budge. Some of them even fall asleep! But if I have to take a skin biopsy, it's suddenly the most painful thing in the world, even if they've been completely numbed. Clearly, motivation for looking good works as anesthesia, while fear of the medical unknown can cause pain. It appears my undergraduate psychology degree continues to play an important role in my practice. But remember: variation in your mood, recent alcohol intake, fatigue, menses, and other factors also can affect pain tolerance.

Find the Right Fit

No matter what medical procedure you're having, you need to feel that you're being cared for. This means you have to have that *click* with your provider. And you have to trust your instincts. A doctor you consult with might have the most glowing recommendations in the world, but if you don't like him or her, it will be difficult to create a trusting and truthful relationship. Sometimes someone's personality just rubs you the wrong way. You don't know why. It just happens. If so, listen to your gut and find someone else.

It's really hard to ever feel happy with someone who doesn't make you feel good.

My biggest accomplishment is not making people look pretty. My biggest accomplishment is making them feel comfortable with me and what I can do for them. Comfort in what I do and comfort in their own skin. Getting a patient to feel comfortable with me is a form of an intimate relationship. Someone is letting me inject things into their face. These injectables are temporary. A patient who is not happy with the results or the practitioner won't come back. That's why trusting your doctor from day one is so important. Only after several visits and trying different procedures will I be able to recommend things that will meet your realistic, aesthetic goals; recognize your tolerance for downtime; be aware of your budget; and have a better sense of who you are.

I always tell my patients that they're not going under the knife and I'm not going to be throwing them into the deep end of the pool. Some patients, for example, come in once a week for little bits until we reach the desired end result. Ultimately, my goal is to get people to come back in several months, sit in my chair, and say, "Okay, Dr. Frank, do what you've got to do." That's my greatest achievement because it means they trust me. They trust my skill, they trust my judgment, and they trust that I'm going to do something that's in their best interest. Aesthetically, safety-wise, and cost-effectively.

> *Enthusiasm is contagious. On the flip side, so is negativity.*

You also will know you're in good hands when it's obvious that your practitioner loves what they're doing. It not only makes you relax but feel good, especially if you're about to get some injections in your face! Enthusiasm is contagious. On the flip side, so is negativity. The doctors I train have many questions about patient care, because they too can believe the erroneous stereotypes about the kind of people who go to cosmetic dermatologists. That these patients are neurotic, demanding, insecure, and impossible to please. Well, I tell these newbie doctors the only cosmetic dermatologists who have patients like that need to take a good hard look in the mirror, because that attitude is all about *them*, not their patients. You attract what you put out in this world.

My patients are not neurotic and impossible to please. Most of them take care of themselves, work very hard, play very hard, do their best to take care of themselves, and connect with their loved ones. They're wonderful, interesting, engaged, and thoughtful people. If they're demanding, it's only because they see these demands as a way to better themselves.

CHAPTER 3

Aestheticians: Treatments and Devices

Nothing in the world can be compared to the human face. It is a land one can never tire of exploring.

—CARL THEODOR DREYER

I love aestheticians, and I respect their very visible talents and the insight and care they provide to all their clients. My practice wouldn't be the same without them. Their skilled hands and rigorous training make them experts in stand-alone skincare, product recommendations, and in providing supportive care for my more intense treatments. They are especially good at helping people deal with issues such as acne, other skin inflammations, and plain old stress. Most important, they spend significant time with their clients over prolonged treatment periods learning about their skin, their personalities, and their individual needs in a way a physician may not have time to do.

Having a treatment done by an experienced and licensed aesthetician should always make you feel good and look even better. But, as with all medical practitioners, there can be problems with some aestheticians who step out of bounds, make false claims, and offer services for which they have no license and substandard training. This is true, as well, of doctors that step out of their training and licensure. In the rapidly expanding world of cosmetic dermatology and aesthetic skin care, there is an enormous and unnecessary turf war going on, not only between doctors and aestheticians, but between doctors of various specialties, nurses, physician assistants, and the wide array of wellness-oriented service providers who all want to sell and perform beauty-enhancement services. Understandably, the competition exists because this sector is the largest and quickest-growing portion of the entire beauty industry.

The only problems that exist are the poor regulation and monitoring of these procedures, and the liability for those performing them outside the confines of their training, experience, and expertise. For this reason, the largest growth in my practice today is managing complications and poor cosmetic outcomes done by others. Your dermatologist, aesthetician, plastic surgeon, nutritionist, trainer, internist, holistic healer, or anyone else should be complementary—not competitive. Always seek providers who know their roles and respect other experts. Steer clear of supposed experts who bad-mouth the value of another's expertise.

I am very fortunate to work quite closely with the incomparable Georgia Louise. As a leader in the skincare industry, she has developed a European-style aesthetician brand of her own over the past twenty years with her team of skincare experts at her atelier in NYC. We speak regularly about our common patients and work to complement and customize our services for them. She has been kind enough to share her insights with us in this chapter.

Christopher Drummond, who provides the information on cosmetic tattooing for this chapter, is an expert cosmetic tattoo artist and one of the first practitioners of microblading in the United States. He is the lead cosmetic tattoo artist for PFRANKMD &

Skin Salon and is the CEO and founder of CD Brows and CD Beauty Cosmetics. I am fortunate to have his expertise for my brand and for this book.

What Aestheticians Can Do

There are very important differences between what aestheticians can legally claim and/or do and what licensed medical professionals do. Although there is significant overlap and state laws can vary and be confusing, the biggest difference is between superficial versus deep treatments and short-term versus long-term results and downtime.

> *Basically, anything that penetrates the more superficial layers of the skin is considered a medical procedure.*

Basically, anything that penetrates the more superficial layers of the skin is considered a medical procedure. If a device requires FDA approval, has more than a few hours of downtime, or carries risks that require informed consent, it's often a treatment that requires a medical professional such as a doctor, nurse, or a physician assistant. They should only provide supportive and complementary care to the treatment of skin disease and the more invasive forms of cosmetic treatments.

So what *can* aestheticians do? They can make you look and feel wonderful, especially if you want immediate results. They can provide soothing, refreshing, and restorative treatments that give you a glow and contribute to healthy and beautiful skin. Examples are:

- Various types of facials that work on the top layers of skin
- Microdermabrasion to exfoliate the dead layers of the epidermis

- Very superficial microneedling
- Ultrasound, electrical stimulation, radiofrequency treatments, cryotherapy, and LED light treatments (which aren't lasers), that affect superficial layers of the dermis and epidermis
- Cosmetic tattooing. It's a needle, but it's superficial
- Massage and lymphatic drainage
- Laser hair removal; in some states, anything laser-oriented other than hair removal is considered a medical procedure
- Recommend over-the-counter skin regimens that are suited to your skin type and lifestyle.

> *It doesn't take many years to acquire an aesthetician license, but it does take many more years, great experience, judgment, and art to become a superior aesthetician practitioner.*

It doesn't take many years to acquire an aesthetician license, but it does take many more years, great experience, judgment, and art to become a *superior* aesthetician practitioner. The bad news is that, with so many options out there, it's difficult to know what might be an effective treatment, what might just be hype, and who to go to. At the very least, aesthetician treatments should always leave you feeling good and seeing some kind of improvement. None of them should be painful—if they are, it's generally a signal that something deeper and riskier is being performed and likely should be put in the hands of a healthcare professional.

Let's take a look at these treatments in more detail.

Facial Basics: An Aesthetician's Perspective

By Georgia Louise, *celebrity facialist*

What This Procedure Is and Conditions It Treats

A lot of dermatologists say, "If you don't need it, why bother to see an aesthetician? I can prevent aging, and they're just massaging your skin and making you hydrated." Well, that might have been true back in the 1980s and 1990s, but guess what: aestheticians are very much at the forefront of skin care, and we spend hours manipulating, massaging, draining, and touching the skin of our clients in a very different way than dermatologists touch and work on skin.

There are, of course, still aestheticians who only do deep cleansing and hydrating facials that come with a massage. These facials are soothing and relaxing, but the aestheticians who do them can't and don't really understand skin anatomy and skin type and skin condition. That's not me! There are so many devices and modalities that aestheticians now have access to. It's not about homing in on what you see on top of the skin; it's about what's causing the skin condition in the first place.

I think coming from Europe, where I got intense training and a master's degree, has helped me over the past twenty years to look at skin and analyze its condition and then be able to figure out which products, machines, and other devices might work best to enhance, tone, and hydrate it. I understand the biology of the skin. The American attitude is becoming more like that in Europe, where people rely on their aestheticians as much as their dermatologists, sometimes more. My clients want natural-looking skin. A client might tell me that she has dry skin, but I can look at it and see the inflammation caused by stress, and then create a regimen that will give results.

That's what aestheticians should do: give you rebalanced, retextured, rehydrated, and healthier-looking skin without the need to do anything invasive involving recovery.

If you're pregnant, sensitive, or if you have an upcoming special event, an aesthetician can help. Whether my client is a famous actress, a model, a professional, or a homemaker, I can give them a glow with an incredible treatment, as well as an instant lift that lasts two weeks. Anyone who has these kinds of treatments will look well-rested and glowing.

My clients come to see me for many different reasons. They want to understand their skin better so they can know how to treat it. And they're coming in for prevention, to get a modality like microcurrent or radiofrequency. A good analogy is that you always brush your teeth at home, but the dentist is where you go for a deep cleaning and treatment. You can maintain your skin with moisturizers and serums and exfoliants and sunscreen, but you come to the aesthetician because it's a deeper all-around experience. Nearly all topical skin conditions are caused by inflammation, and what is the number-one trigger for inflammation? Stress. A good aesthetician understands that and can leave the client feeling calm and relaxed, even for just the hour—but this sets them up for the whole week. Facials are all about creating an experience that's calming, soothing, and de-stressing. The effective high-tech devices I use are just one area of the magic. That's why I don't call what I do just "facials." They're transformative treatments.

After a facial, you should always be able to go straight out for dinner. You'll get compliments on your skin that night and when you wake up in the morning. That's the beauty of it.

What It Can't Do

Even the best facials can't give you permanent results, although your skin will look better the more often you have them.

Pros/Cons

If you're young and your skin is healthy, then you can have a facial when you like. But after about the age of twenty-six or so, your skin starts to change as the collagen begins to become depleted and less elastic, and that's when we start to talk about prevention and anti-aging products. At that point, bimonthly should be enough. When you get into your thirties and up, ideally, you should have a monthly facial. That's when skin cell turnover start to slow down, and you need more intense exfoliation to get rid of the dead skin cells. If your budget allows, a facial every week will have noticeable anti-aging effects.

For the best and safest results, you need to go to a licensed med-spa such as Dr. Frank's, or an established salon with aestheticians like myself who've been properly trained to use the modalities and devices. I'm never going to put a laser near a face; never go to an aesthetician for a laser. They scare me because it's literally a weapon in the wrong hands, and I've seen treatments go wrong and cause serious damage. I refer my clients to colleagues like Dr. Frank, who has the training and knows precisely which laser to use for whatever specific condition and skin tone. Aestheticians don't know that.

You deserve to have a quality treatment, so do your homework beforehand. Your expectations won't be unrealistic and you'll be happier with the results. Ask questions like: What machines and devices do you have? What frequencies? Where were you trained? What are your credentials? How long have you been using these devices? What are the potential side effects? What kind of products are you using? What brand is it? Is it professional strength? It takes a lot of education, licensing, and time for the best aestheticians to get where they are.

Treatments During Facials

Chemical Peels

What This Procedure Is and Conditions It Treats

Superficial chemical exfoliation works to boost collagen, help skin-cell turnover, and improve simple maladies of color and tone in the skin (such as unevenness, blotchiness, or hyperpigmentation spots). Light peels usually last for one to two months, and people tend to buy a series of four to six monthly treatments. They're often part of a comprehensive facial.

What It Can't Do

Peels are best for superficial wrinkles and exfoliation. They can't remove deeper wrinkles or provide toning and tightening to improve sagging.

Pros/Cons

Aestheticians can't perform medium or deep peels which, of course, have much more effective results. With peels, it's no pain, no gain!

LED Light

What This Procedure Is and Conditions It Treats

LED stands for light-emitting diode, and this treatment uses various wavelengths of light that heat the skin for different skin issues. Primarily, red is used for collagen and elastin boosting and for fine lines and wrinkles; blue is for acne zapping and to reduce excess oil production; amber is good for redness reduction and broken capillaries; green is to deal with pigmentation issues; and yellow and white are for reducing inflammation.

What It Can't Do

The light isn't as potent as lasers and doesn't penetrate deeply, so some people see little to no effect.

Pros/Cons

Georgia Louise: LED treatments are usually used in addition to other treatments. Basically, you lie down with your eyes protected and let the lights shine on your face for fifteen to twenty minutes. They're a gentle and painless way to make your skin feel brighter and clearer. I'm mainly multi-tasking when I use light therapy— my clients will get light for twenty minutes with me manipulating or massaging the products that will penetrate into the derma layer of their skin.

Lymphatic Drainage

What This Procedure Is and Conditions It Treats

This is a medical massage that can improve skin appearance by improving circulation of the lymphatic system. It can help with inflammation, reduce puffiness, and brighten the skin to help give you a bit of a glow, and is often done as part of a facial.

What It Can't Do

Lymphatic drainage is a temporary treatment, so it needs to be done regularly to see or feel any results. It can't make a permanent change in your circulatory system.

Pros/Cons

There's really no downside to the treatment. Always be sure to massage upward, as your lymphatic vessels drain downwards, thanks to gravity.

Microcurrent

What This Procedure Is and Conditions It Treats

Microcurrent is a technique using two wands of a device that emits a very low-voltage electrical current to stimulate and tone your facial muscles. (It was originally used as a medical device to help improve paralyzed facial muscles.) It can help slightly lift muscles, reduce puffiness, and is touted as being able to stimulate collagen and elastin production.

What It Can't Do

Although there is no data proving its effectiveness as a cosmetic treatment, microcurrent is touted as a "'non-facelift' facelift." It can be temporarily effective, but it can't tighten and tone the way lasers or surgery can.

Pros/Cons

Georgia Louise: In the last five years, microcurrent treatments have been in high demand, and there have been many improvements to the technology, so some of my clients have a lifting and tightening effect that can last up to two weeks. I do half the face and show my client the mirror and they're like, "Ohmigod, it's lifted now!" It's painless and safe, and it provides a relaxing massage (great for lymphatic drainage) but can be a bit tingly. I believe that if you do it regularly every few weeks, your muscles change due to the stimulation, and the tightening effect lasts longer. The more you do it over time, the better and longer-lasting the results. The downside to this is that if you stop the treatments, the muscles go back to where they were.

Microdermabrasion

What This Procedure Is and Conditions It Treats

Using a device that sprays tiny crystals on the face, microdermabrasion is a gentle and effective physical exfoliation, similar to a light chemical peel, to remove sun damage, light wrinkles, acne scars, and a dull complexion. It is often done as part of a facial.

What It Can't Do

Because this procedure only exfoliates the topmost skin layers, it can't remove lines, wrinkles, or scars.

Pros/Cons

This is a procedure that might leave you a little pink or bruised afterwards, but it should be gentle and give you a clearer and more even skin tone, especially if you haven't exfoliated in a while. It can be helpful if you have enlarged pores, as it will get the gunk out. But because it's gentle, you should have gentle expectations!

Radiofrequency

What This Procedure Is and Conditions It Treats

Radiofrequency treatments noninvasively boost collagen levels and improve elasticity, tightening, and toning of the skin. They work by heating the skin tissue, which tightens the collagen fibers and stimulates more collagen and elastin production. There can be minor swelling, bruising, and redness for a day afterward. You usually need several sessions to see results.

What It Can't Do

Aesthetician radiofrequency sessions, although effective, can't treat skin as aggressively as a dermatologist can. More treatments are thus required to see desired results. The power level of the machines an aesthetician uses is different, as is the manner of which the energy is delivered and flows through the body. The simple rule is: if it hurts at all, then it is potent and deep enough that it requires a medical professional to perform it. It also isn't a good option for people whose facial skin is significantly loose and sagging, as more invasive tightening procedures are needed. It is, however, great for maintenance of skin tone during facials.

Pros/Cons

Georgia Louise: I call radiofrequency treatments my face iron. They're like a massage and are very quick. The machine is not as strong or powerful as lasers, but it's safer without creating too much irritation or redness.

Ultrasound

What This Procedure Is and Conditions It Treats

Similar to radiofrequency treatments, ultrasound uses heat to noninvasively boost collagen levels and improve elasticity, tightening, and toning of the skin.

What It Can't Do

See Radiofrequency.

Pros/Cons

Georgia Louise: Ultrasound allows the treatment products to better penetrate into your skin and will give you a nice glow. I tell my clients it's like having an IV directly into your skin.

Cosmetic Tattooing/Microblading

By Christopher Drummond, *master cosmetic tattoo artist*

What This Procedure Is and Conditions It Treats—Christopher's Perspective

Cosmetic tattooing can be done for various cosmetic or medical purposes, such as scar revision, discoloration, nipple reconstruction after a mastectomy, vitiligo, or alopecia. Wonders can be done for cosmetic issues that are resistant to cosmetic dermatology treatments, such as lasers, or are not cost-effective with other treatments. This is common in the case of white scars such as facelift and breast-lift scars, stretch marks, or loss of pigmentation anywhere on the body, including the lips. Most commonly, it's done to thicken or color in eyebrows, especially for those who have hair loss. Most of the pigments used are plant-based, so the colors are more natural. (Regular body tattoos tend to use synthetic pigments and a stronger machine, which make them very hard to remove, even with lasers.) The difference between cosmetic tattooing and microblading has to do with the instruments used. Tattooing uses a needle and a machine; microblading uses a hand tool with between five to twenty-one tiny needles to apply the color into your skin. For eyebrows, you'll usually need two two-hour sessions.

What It Can't Do

Cosmetic tattooing can't undo any damage done or stimulate new hair growth—only disguise the areas with pigment. It is also semi-permanent; it gradually fades and won't last longer than one to three years.

Pros/Cons

When done properly to hide hair loss, the tattoos look remarkably like real hair. I work with a lot of people who have a hypothyroid condition which makes them lose the end part of their brow, and they're very embarrassed and upset when they only have half a brow or very light brows. I can't tell you how many women have told me that cosmetic tattooing has literally changed their lives.

Since the pigments eventually fade, this is good if you're not happy with the results, but bad if you're happy with the results. Touch-ups can be performed for maintenance.

Microblading has gotten very popular, but it is totally unregulated in the United States—which means that basically anyone can take a three-hour online course and call themselves a trained technician. Body tattoo artists must have a several-year apprenticeship where they are not permitted to do any work on real people, but microblading has no such requirements. Bad results can look very fake and way too dark for your skin tone. A skilled tattoo artist can work wonders, but you need a lot of experience to do it well, as everyone's skin is different—and complications can occur. Never go to anyone who hasn't had years of training, and make sure the artist has a relationship with a dermatologist to manage any medical skin issues related to the treatment.

The field of cosmetic tattooing remains exciting and continues to grow with new procedures and techniques. Lip blushing, which restores youthful pinkness in the lips, and BB Glow, which microneedles temporary makeup into the skin, are just two of the exciting new technologies on the horizon.

CHAPTER 4

Medical and Professional Treatments and Devices

There is no exquisite beauty...without some
strangeness in the proportion.

—EDGAR ALLEN POE

Not that long ago, a wellness guru and teacher in her forties, known for her expertise with naturopathic treatments, came to see me. She was in great shape and looked fantastic, but time catches up with our skin, no matter how well we take care of ourselves.

"I can't believe I'm sitting here, considering putting filler in my face or getting zapped by a laser," she said as I looked at her information form and saw that she wanted help for hyperpigmentation issues and wrinkles. I also saw that she'd been using prescription-strength creams, gone to different aestheticians, had platelet-rich plasma injections (more on that later), and many sessions of acupuncture to treat the dark circles under her eyes—a treatment which left her with nothing but black eyes for a week every single time.

"Listen, the most important choice that you have here is your choice to do nothing," I told her. "You're beautiful, you look great, you take fantastic care of yourself, and I'm sure, even though this may be an insecure moment now, that you're a pretty positive person. That's how people perceive you. But I'm here to change your misconceptions about what getting filler is and about what getting laser is, because they don't have to be scary. And, most important, I'm going to show you that, except for all that amazing self-care, all those treatments you did before were a waste of time and money. So I want you to walk out of here saying one of two things: 'I'm going to live with it,' or, 'I'm going to take the right steps with the right expert to do things that are going to make me look better and feel better.'"

I promised her either choice would be okay. I don't want anyone to tell themselves, "Oh, what am I doing to myself with this cosmetic procedure and why am I putting toxins in my body? If you make the choice to do the procedures, I'm very confident that you're going to come out with a newfound respect and lack of fear about them.

Then I told her, "I'm going to teach you just like you teach your students." That's when I saw her visibly relax.

This patient was a perfect example of the type of reeducation that I do every day. Although she had wasted all that time, energy, and money for years, none of the treatments she'd gotten had *harmed* her, but they hadn't worked either. They did, however, cost money, involved physical trauma and recovery, and, most important, wasted invested faith in the belief that she was being delivered something that would make her feel better about something that bothered her visually—which obviously had a significant emotional impact on her. And, while some of my treatments might create similar trauma, I guarantee you, when all is said and done, she's most likely going to look much, much better!

So I want you to use this chapter as *your* reeducation filter about cosmetic medical procedures. It's just human nature to want one magic bullet, one pill, one answer—and that's not going to happen! We all want to seek out the most natural, least-invasive, safest, and quickest means to satisfy any goal, cosmetic or aesthetic. But this is not always the most effective approach. The most important thing I can do for any patient is to be honest, be empathic, provide choices, and essentially give them a no-bullshit direction based on my twenty years of experience.

Sadly, by the time many people get in my chair, they have learned that just because a procedure exists doesn't mean it works...and even if it does work, it doesn't mean it works for everybody. There's no such thing as satisfaction guaranteed when it comes to rejuvenation of any kind. Beware of anyone that says something has zero risk or works for everyone. Nothing, whether it's putting on a new moisturizer or getting Botox or starting a new workout regimen, is without physical or emotional risk. The best way to protect yourself is to arm yourself with knowledge and find a provider that you can trust knows your goals and expectations, so you can minimize risk.

How to Prioritize Medical Treatments

During my patient consultation, I find out what their concerns are, help them target them, and figure out what treatments will make the biggest difference. Obviously, as you know, this will not be the same for everybody, which is why I offer so many devices, injectables, and procedures. I have over thirty-five different devices alone, four that work only on pigment issues and four more that work only on skin tightening. I also have fifteen different injectables. I have quick fixes, long-term fixes that require multiple visits, and more. I'm also often asked if I do the same procedures and devices on men as I do on women, or if I do the same for seniors as I do for millennials. My answer is that I often use the same technology on every generation, on every gender, and on every ethnicity. It's not *which* treatment I do that's so different. It's *how* I do it and the psychological intent behind it. All these treatments are instruments in a symphony. Of course you want the best quality of instruments, but, ultimately, it is how they are played that makes all the difference. Different scores being played, varying audiences, concert halls, solos, or duets. All instruments choreographed in variable arrangements to make the sounds, the impressions, and the results we desire. This is the art of aesthetic rejuvenation.

So when asked by patients, "How do you know what to do or what to choose for me?" I tell them it will take my ten years of training followed by my twenty years of experience to know the best step-by-step treatment for each individual.

Choosing Treatment Techniques: By Safety, Efficacy/Expectations, Short- or Long-term Effect, Downtime, and Cost

I've said it before, and I'll say it again: safety always comes first. Smokers, for example, will have more risk in healing for certain procedures than nonsmokers. People on blood thinners bleed more. Darker-skinned patients have some degree of elevated risk with certain types of lasers.

My job is to not just deliver the best choice and the best quality of procedure, but to prioritize concerns with the greatest safety, *then* the greatest results. Followed by the greatest cost advocacy. All while keeping in mind the lifestyle issues that will affect your choice as well as your skin color, skin condition, and any other medical issues.

Safety always comes first.

Next on the discussion list is checking off the things you *don't* need. Throughout my youth, while navigating life's innumerous choices, my father would repeatedly reinforce his view of optimizing outcomes by telling me to remember the rule of KISS: Keep It Simple, Stupid! Many patients like to start with one simple procedure, like neuromodulator wrinkle relaxers (e.g., Botox), and prefer to be eased into other treatments. Some want to go as deep and invasive as possible from day one.

The bottom line: we have wonder treatments, but there is no manual. And there are plenty of situations, such as scars or wrinkles on people with a certain lifestyle, budget, or other factors, where I can't help at all.

In fact, most of the issues I treat can't be gotten rid of. When someone comes in for injectables, I can often make the wrinkles overwhelmingly better, but I can't get rid of them entirely. When I use the most aggressive lasers on wrinkles, I can make them better, but I can't get rid of them. So it's a big red flag when a patient says, "I want to get rid of this. I want these *gone.*" I tell them that I *can't* do that, but I *can* make significant improvements, giving them guidelines based on what I'm absorbing of their psychological expectations, while explaining that I'm selling them something that is really in their best interest aesthetically.

Just remember, when evaluating your options, that no one needs ten of them—but you should be offered several. There is no one solution or option for any cosmetic concern. It must be appropriate, as you know by now, for your age, your skin color, your skin type, your budget, and, more than anything else, your expectations.

The most efficient way to discuss options is in terms of the level of the skin being treated. For example, if you have pigment issues, resurfacing devices treat the upper layers of the skin. For wrinkles and scars, problems tend to be in the mid to deep dermis, where collagen and elastin are found, where the sun damage is, and where the loss of elasticity happens. In the deepest level, there's the fat layer, which is all about volume restoration or depletion.

In addition, there are options within each category. As you'll see in this chapter, there are many kinds of fillers. Some are reversible, and others are not. The ones that last the longest are irreversible, so it's up to you and your practitioner to decide on the level of risk you're comfortable with. If you're anxious about the results, for instance, a reversible filler is likely to be your best option until you're more comfortable with the procedure. It may be worth it to you to pay the higher cost of that filler.

Once I've pinpointed the issues, then I can move on to specifics that meet the patient's nonmedical needs, such as downtime, cost, and other lifestyle issues, because we're talking about elective procedures that make subjective differences.

Let's say someone is unhappy with the smoker's lines above her lip. I will explain that the best *result* is not necessarily the best *treatment* for them. That's because the best result would be aggressive laser resurfacing. It works extremely well but it has a lot of downtime (no sun exposure at all for at least a month), some risks, and is expensive. A lot of patients are not going to want to invest that amount of trauma and energy, and they feel it's too invasive. Or they're outdoors people and can't stay indoors for several weeks. Others assume that Botox or similar products will work, but they don't know that they're only effective for a very specific group—those who, when they talk or are at rest or sleeping, are constantly pursing their lips. Botox works for them because their lines are caused by a muscle issue. However, Botox may be totally wrong for someone who is a professional wind-instrument player or who likes to drink out of straws, because it would weaken the mouth muscles ever so slightly. As a result, about 75 percent of the time, fillers are the best option.

For those on a budget, there are almost always a number of treatments in the same category for many common cosmetic issues. I usually direct them first toward the simplest things that make the biggest differences. Botox or one of the other neuro-modulators tends to be the first gateway drug. The reason why Botox is a household name is because it's an exemplary treatment, where there's a huge bang for your buck, a low rate of dissatisfaction, and a very large safety profile. And no, just because it can be poisonous in other forms in nature under other circumstances does not mean you are injecting "poison" per se into your body. Most things in nature can be lifesaving and beneficial in one reality and totally destructive in another. This is the paradox of life, science, and particularly medicine, time and time again.

Different Treatments Have Overlap with Each Other

You will notice in the Basic Procedures section that some categories have overlap. Resurfacing treatments can tackle wrinkles, for example, and so can muscle modification and volume optimization. This is why I often combine different treatments and devices for the same problem. For frown lines, I'd start with Botox. For marionette lines near the lips, I'd start with a filler. For deeper lines, I'd use a laser or a combination of the above. It all depends on your unique factors, such as your age and your skin's elasticity, the severity of the issue, the variable ways to improve the problem, and your willingness to pursue its improvement. I always say to patients that the greatest way to get the best and most natural-appearing results is to combine several small things rather than to do a lot of one thing. Combination treatments always lead to several subtle but overall significant results.

> *Combination treatments always lead to several subtle but overall significant results.*

How to Know Which Treatments to Combine

I generally start with simplest and most straightforward. For many, these are injectables or quick-fix lasers, whether for the face or anywhere on the body. After that, other devices come into play that may require several treatments or may have some downtime, whether for tightening, wrinkling, scarring, or any malady of cosmetic concern. Always try the most straightforward procedure first, then consider, if at all, adding other supplemental things that could help the situation, including not only procedures, but lifestyle changes. Of course, when I'm treating sun damage and wrinkles, patients start to consider for the first time their issues of sun exposure. Or, when they are treating problems of volume, too much or too little, they think about their nutritional lifestyle, and so on. This is all part of the pro-aging playbook—thinking beyond one answer to any problem.

What the Basic Procedures and Devices Can Do

The categories in this section cover the basic procedures and devices and explain how they work.

Botox and Other Neuromodulators

In the new millennium, botulinum toxin type A became the first revolutionary product to inaugurate the global quick-fix mentality of modern cosmetic dermatology. In doing so, it smoothened out facial wrinkles throughout the world and launched thousands of sitcom jokes, memes, and the prospects of easily accessible, safe, effective, and a profitable fountain of youth. It has literally and figuratively changed the face of my medical field and was just getting its footing in society's vernacular while I was in my dermatology residency program in the late 1990s.

Botox has proven to be an enormous gateway to cosmetic injectables, as it's so quick and easy to the outside observer—and it works. It's, by far, the most popular procedure in cosmetic dermatology. When done well, Botulinum toxin is an amazing pro-aging rejuvenator. The key word here, of course, is *well*. As with all new and fabulous things, society has a tendency to over-indulge. And, yes, there is too much of a good thing. Too much Botox can cause the opposite of pro-aging, making people look unnaturally smooth, fake, and *older* than they are. Here's how *not* to look that way.

How Botox Works

Botox is the brand name for botulinum toxin type A, a drug in the neuromodulator category. Neuromodulators are substances that chemically interfere with acetylcholine, a common neurotransmitter, at nerve/muscle junctions. It prevents nerve cells in the muscles from being able to communicate with each other, which can augment muscle function and stretch out the wrinkles, formed by normal expressions over time. There are over a dozen different neuromodulators on the market throughout the world, and in addition to Botox, those most commonly used in the US are Dysport, Xeomin, and Jeuveau. Other products with small clinical differences continue to be in the research pipeline.

Botulinum toxin is a protein derived from the bacteria *Clostridium botulinum*, which can cause the deadly paralytic disease botulism and is considered one of the most toxic materials in the world. It was first isolated in the 1940s and has been used clinically to treat muscular problems of the eye since the 1970s. It was originally discovered to have the potential for cosmetic uses in the late 1980s by a Canadian ophthalmologist and dermatologist couple, Alastair and Jean Carruthers. Their groundbreaking research helped pave the way for Botox to go from the experimental vanity of those in the know during the 1990s to its subsequent

FDA approval to treat glabellar lines (frown lines between your eyes) in 2002. This in turn led to a spike in direct-to-consumer marketing and a new era of how the world views cosmetic rejuvenation.

It is one of the most studied and used chemical compounds in the world, and now 50 percent of its use, both FDA-approved and off-label, is for non-cosmetic medical purposes such as migraine headaches, neck and eye spasms, teeth grinding, excessive sweating, bladder disorder, anal fissures, neuropathic pain, chronic pain, cerebral palsy, and even depression and the treatment of keloid scars.

Botox can't really kill you. There is no appreciable danger in using neuromodulators, as they are highly diluted, purified, and only applied locally in minuscule doses, not systemically, but some of my patients getting it for the first time are still very wary. "I'm worried about Botox because I don't want botulism," they tell me. "I don't want anything toxic in my body."

If so, I ask them if they've ever taken aspirin, or had an alcoholic drink, or smoked something, or just breathed city air. Those are potentially "toxic" substances that can easily kill us, but we don't think about them that way.

The other understandable comment I get is, "I don't believe in Botox." My answer is always that it's fine. No one has to believe in Santa either, but trust me—Botox exists! Although it's not for everyone. it happens to be one of the simplest, safest, cost- and time-effect treatments to help turn back the clock. It has also stood the test of time.

The greatest misconception about any cosmetic treatment, particularly neuromodulators, is the fear of looking obvious and fake. Although some people want that fake look, most don't, and certainly not my patients. I tell my patients that they're only noticing the bad work out there. They can't tell the good work because they just think those people look great!

Botox Works Best For...

Neuromodulators have numerous uses cosmetically. Botox can remove the deep crease between your eyes, eradicate crow's feet, forehead lines, dimpling in the chin, and fine lines around the lips. It can help lift the neck and jawline lines by relaxing certain muscles in the region. It can thin out the width of the face by treating the muscles of chewing, and smooth your skin texture by placing Botox in the top layers of skin, preventing new lines from forming. It can even be injected into the tip of the nose to give it a mini-lift.

The most common reason that people are getting treatment now is prevention. The largest growth is with young people who develop early signs of wrinkling in their twenties or by their early thirties. Small amounts of "Baby Botox" go a long way for these patients to erase what they have and prevent progression.

When I was a resident in the 1990s at NYU Langone Medical Center, Botox was not yet FDA-approved for cosmetic use, but people were using it off-label. Only the cosmetically conscious were aware of this secret anti-wrinkle drug of the rich and famous. So I tried it. At twenty-seven, I had lines in my forehead. They didn't bother me much, but what did at twenty-seven? Once the lines were erased, I was overwhelmed, as most first-timers are, with the efficacy and ease of the treatment. My peers thought I was crazy to continue using it once it wore off. "You're too young to do Botox," they told me. "You don't need it! This will be used only on older patients when approved." It was then I saw the forest through the trees. Now, at fifty, with twenty-three years of neuromodulator use behind me—me and my close-to-wrinkle-free forehead—I'm glad I didn't listen to any of my peers. Pro-aging starts young. It's always easier to clean up your room when it's not too dirty!

Avoid Botox If...

Neuromodulators don't work for certain anatomies, or if age or skin conditions have caused the wrinkles to become too entrenched. Botox may minimize a deep wrinkle, but if the result is negligible or its effect depends on dramatically affecting the natural motion of your face, it is probably best to consider other procedures such as fillers, lasers, or plastic surgery. As neuromodulators augment muscle movement and therefore can alter the shapes of features, they can sometimes flatten the eyebrows or pull them up too high. This is where the skill and the judgment of the injector play the most important role. Sadly, the ease of the treatment gives the false impression that everyone is a candidate and anything is possible.

For a lot of people, neuromodulators are not the answer, as they will do something to the mobility of the face that will make the person unhappy, particularly if they are in the arts. Many of my patients tell me that they don't care if their face falls off—they just want those wrinkles gone. Some, however, are more precise. I had a patient who was a very expressive thirty-five-year-old, and happy with a little bit of Botox around her eyes. She desperately wanted to treat some small wrinkles on her forehead but not decrease the full range of expression in her upper face. I told her that very small injections would make a difference, but it would be impossible not to alter her expression at all—it's those expressions that were causing the wrinkles. There simply was no way to predict how she would look, so I advised her against treatment because I knew that even a minuscule injection would have left her upset.

I also tell actors and comedians, especially those with very expressive faces, that it may not be worth doing. Their ability to show emotions is essential to their careers and persona. No one wants to see Meryl Streep look frozen.

How It's Done

Botulinum toxin comes in freeze-dried powder form and is reconstituted with a sterile saline solution so it can then be injected through a fine needle. It has to be used soon after reconstitution or it can lose much of its effectiveness. Beware providers that aren't performing the procedure all day—old product is not as strong!

Pain Scale and Recuperation

Botox is one of the least painful injections, and, as you'll just feel a little pinch or burning sensation. There's no need for topical numbing beforehand. Sometimes a vibratory device is an effective distraction. I often use that with a bit of "talkesthesia."

You might see a slight bruising or a tiny bit of swelling, but most people have no reaction whatsoever and go right back to whatever they were doing before their injections. The fluid bump gets absorbed in ten to fifteen minutes. You don't want to manipulate the area for an hour or two afterward (no facials, please!), but you don't have to worry about walking around like a robot with your head held up high for a few hours, which is what patients used to be told. It's okay to bend over or lean over cautiously if you drop something!

When You'll See Results

It usually takes about two to ten days to see Botox's full effect, depending on the brand and on the patient. You need to give it seven to ten days.

Side Effects

Other than local side effects like bruising and swelling, physiological side effects are rare. True allergies are not seen to botulinum toxin itself. There are patients who can get a headache or temporary flu-like symptoms. Overall, Botox is a remarkably tolerable drug. Most of the potential side effects are cosmetic, commonly caused if the drug is injected too near or shifts to a muscle you don't want weakened. Very rarely, there can be drooping of the upper eyelid itself, which can be treated with eye drops until its own resolution. The brow can also look too heavy or there can be unnatural changes of the shape of the eyebrow; if so, slight adjustments with strategically placed injections can be made.

There is the problematic side effect when too much Botox is used, leaving a person looking unnaturally smooth, fake, and plastic. Some people are so fearful of wrinkles that they overdo it. It is essential the first time you try Botox to give feedback to your provider. Adjustments can be made. I always say I would rather touch up a patient for free than overdo something. About 10 percent of my patients require these touch-ups occasionally, and the conversation about what or how we are going to achieve the best cosmetic results is essential. It's an art form, and no two treatments are exactly alike.

How Long It Lasts

In general, Botox doesn't last more than three to six months. It's impossible to predict this exactly, although some patients have told me that it *seems* to last longer if they see me regularly. Patients also comment how the wrinkles never seem to go back to their original severity. This is often proven when women take a "Botox break" due to pregnancy and breastfeeding. Botox and babies are not a good mix!

The lack of longevity is unfortunate for those who love it, but not so unfortunate for anyone who isn't happy with their practitioner, as Botox can't be undone (as some fillers can). New brands arrive with various longevities, but there is still no perfect brand. I often use all of the available neuromodulators throughout my day, often mixing more than one brand on a single individual. Each product has slightly different characteristics—like differing shades of the same color paint—in time of onset, lasting effect, potency, and diffusion capacity, among others.

I also don't think it would be a good idea to have permanent neuromodulators, as your face is dynamic and always changing over time, and the last thing you'd want to do is commit to permanently altering its muscle activity. Its demands and aesthetics do change over the years—and so should your options for rejuvenation.

What Smart Consumers Know

Because neuromodulators need to be mixed before each use, an unscrupulous practitioner can over-dilute the dose so it's less effective—charging you the same for a procedure that now costs them less. It is impossible to confirm exactly what dose you are getting. If you see the treatment advertised for significantly less than what other practitioners are charging, you can assume you are getting less. These are expensive drugs for providers, not just patients.

As discussed earlier, neuromodulators also need a skilled hand for maximum results. Any MD can legally give you the injections, and so can nurses, dentists, and physician assistants, but that doesn't mean you want them all to do it. Walk-in med spas offer this drug, as well as other cosmetic injectables, and you need to make sure that you will be treated by a healthcare professional who has the experience, the appropriate licensure, and the training to not only make you look good, but to handle complications, rare as they may be.

There is no one injection technique that will work on everyone. Injecting this drug is a delicate art, as it involves inhibiting certain muscles and enhancing certain features without limiting facial expression. The musculature of every face is a bit different, so I am never cavalier about using neuromodulators, as simple as they seem. Problems tend to arise when someone is complacent about technique; like with my toughest cases, I remain duly focused so that things rarely do go wrong. And there's not a week that goes by that I'm not learning new things about what I've been doing successfully for twenty years.

Resurfacing, Rejuvenation, and Smoothing

This category covers procedures for: sun damage, dull or ruddy skin, pigmentation issues, irregular skin texture, scar revision, superficial skin tightening, vascular issues, and fine wrinkles.

The primary treatments are lasers and light-source devices, microneedling, and chemical peels. These sources have become my mainstay for allowing the skin to recharge and repair. For better or worse, there are dozens of devices to choose from, both in the nature of the treatment and the brands that are available.

It is important to note that there is a lot of redundancy in the cosmetic market, as there are often several brands that make similar devices. Make sure that your provider explains the nature of the technology, not just the brand. Often, like the word "Botox"—which is thrown around like the word "Kleenex"—often linguistically represents a category of several products that do similar things. (In other words, Botox is the brand name for a specific neuromodulator.) This also happens with the brand Fraxel, which was the first fractional-laser resurfacing device offering a more novel and safer way to resurface skin about twelve to fifteen years ago. Now, several brands have followed suit with their own variation of the theme. There *are* differences—like the difference between a Ferrari and a Hyundai—and it's important to know what you're getting.

When I talk about skin-resurfacing procedures, I often metaphorically compare them to fixing damaged or worn roads. Depending on the defect in the road, you can choose a technique to fix it. There are occasional potholes to fill or bumps in the road to reduce. But when we need to repave the road, that's what resurfacing devices can do—make a global improvement by removing the old and replacing it with new. The body's amazing healing mechanisms and the skin's unique and rapid cell turnover enable us to do this safely and effectively.

Chemical Peels

How Chemical Peels Work

Before laser resurfacing became as refined and specific as it is today, chemical peels were the mainstay to "repave the road" and rejuvenate. But they also destroy everything in their path. The stronger the acid, the deeper the penetration, as it basically removes skin layers with various agents of potency from the top down. So if you want to target superficial dermal issues, you have to remove the epidermis to do so. The deeper you go, the longer the recovery, the less predictable the course of treatment, and the higher rate of complications.

Chemical Peels Work Best For...

Skin resurfacing. They have proven the test of time in various degrees.

Avoid Chemical Peels If...

If you are of darker skin tones, generally avoid peels that have any downtime.

How They're Done

A chemical solution of varying strength is applied after sterilization and degreasing of the skin. Some chemical peels are time-dependent, while others rely on the number of layers placed.

Pain Scale and Recuperation

Mild to significant, depending on strength.

When You'll See Results

Because all skin resurfacing relies on the body's healing capacity, it generally takes three to five days to see results from mild peels and one week to one month for deeper ones.

Side Effects

All resurfacing techniques incur small risks of infection, poor healing, and pigmentation changes—either too much or too little.

How Long They Last

Peels, along with other resurfacing techniques, are additive and make cumulative changes. The deeper peels are most impactful, unlike injectables, which wear off.

What Smart Consumers Know

One of the reasons I don't regularly perform peels in my office is their lack of versatility and predictability. People respond differently to different types of chemical peels. Also, these agents don't penetrate the skin equally, depending on variables in the uppermost layers. I generally prefer to make cosmetic improvements without creating an open wound. Despite their benefit and widespread use, I generally find chemical peels to be a cheaper form of cosmetic resurfacing, literally and figuratively. Although peels are more cost-effective, there are lasers targeting more specific aspects of the skin that provide tightening effects that peels do not.

Peels are beneficial and, in the right instance, a good alternative for patients on a budget. Fortunately, the days of deep chemical peels are over. They were simply too hard to control and caused too many complications. What you should try do instead is use safe, low-concentration at-home peels (lactic or glycolic acid are good options) and save up for much more aggressive and safer technologies.

Microneedling

Microneedling is a technique that's actually been around for decades. It's gotten a resurgence now because of its ability to be combined with other technologies.

How It Works

Groups of tiny sterile microneedles puncture and wound the skin at various depths. The basis for most cosmetic rejuvenation has to do with promoting controlled damage of the skin to stimulate regrowth of healthy tissue—relying on the skin's rapid and amazing healing mechanisms by getting rid of the old and stimulating the new.

Microneedling Works Best For...

Microneedling can puncture the skin at the various depths that you may want to target. This stimulates collagen and elasticity with subsequent improvements in tightening and texture.

Avoid Microneedling If...

If anyone tells you this is safe to do at home, don't believe them. Despite the availability of home devices, I would avoid them, as this is a medical procedure with risks of bleeding and infection. It requires a sterile environment and professional hands.

How It's Done

Microneedling can be delivered on a stamping or roller-like applicator, usually with groups of needles that puncture the skin at various depths.

Pain Scale and Recuperation

Mild to significant. Superficial treatments feel benign. Deeper treatments require pain management.

When You'll See Results
Within one to four weeks.

Side Effects
Because this procedure creates an open wound, the largest risk is of infection. Precautions and appropriate posttreatment skin care must be taken.

How Long It Lasts
The results are permanent.

What Smart Consumers Know
Microneedling is a relatively controlled benign treatment with a lot of versatility. It has proven to be a novel treatment for scars and superficial skin tightening, particularly for darker skin types that may not tolerate light-based technologies. Although there are a lot of combination treatments available on the market that show enormous promise and advancement, other treatments remain more fad than substance.

Lasers and Light Sources
I love lasers, and I've got dozens in my office. In the new millennium, these technologies took off, allowing us to treat the skin in ways we never could before. There are so many different lasers now that they can treat a wide range of concerns with stunning accuracy.

How Lasers and Light Sources Work
This is a topic that could take days to explain! Lasers and pulsed-light devices are basically fancy, high-tech knives that use various wavelengths of light to produce heat targeting various aspects of the skin. Without going into the intricacies of laser physics,

by varying physical properties of light such as the specific wavelength, the length of the pulses, the depth of penetration, and other parameters, lasers have transformed the field of aesthetic medicine.

First-generation "ablative" lasers that were extremely aggressive came on the market many decades ago. They left a significant open wound that would be so red and raw you'd have to hide in your house for weeks afterward. They effectively removed layers of skin in ways similar to chemical peels—from the top down. They had home-run results on the right patients, but they had extended downtime, painful recoveries, and some risk. They were clearly not for the mainstream.

Thankfully, they have been replaced by innumerable types of improved devices, particularly fractional lasers and lighter-pulsed, multi-wavelength devices, which deliver energy in a manner that can maximize the benefit while decreasing downtime and improving the safety profile. One of the best-known of these is Fraxel, which introduced us to what we call non-ablative fractional resurfacing. This category of devices, which remains the gold standard for many types of laser and non-laser treatments, has the ability to induce skin improvement without creating an open wound like its predecessors. By delivering controlled trauma in a pixelated manner throughout various controlled depths of skin, the columns of heat are staggered in between untreated areas on a microscopic level. This in turn leads to quicker recoveries and safer results for all skin types.

Lasers and Light Sources Work Best For...

More superficial and medium-depth issues of sun damage, texture, superficial scars, and wrinkles. This is mostly because light, in most cases, cannot penetrate so deeply without causing significant damage.

Avoid Lasers and Light Sources If...

If you're tanned, very dark-skinned, have diseases or illnesses, or take medicines that make you light-sensitive, avoid these treatments. There are exceptions to every rule, and there are options for using certain light-based devices with patients that can't necessarily use others.

Pain Scale and Recuperation

This depends entirely on which laser is used. Hair removal feels no more painful than a rubber band snap (if that). When I talk about lasers, it's all about the spectrum of downtime—there's always going to be greater recovery if you're seeking greater results per treatment. Lasers that have more downtime will have the best results. Lasers that require the least downtime may require more treatments.

When You'll See Results

In general, the results often have more to do with the inherent healing and natural turnover of skin cells. Obviously, age plays a role. When removing brown spots, for example, it could take three days in young individuals and one week in someone over sixty-five. Seeing results often relies more on the patient than the technology.

Side Effects

The stronger the laser, the more you will have side effects, such as redness, peeling, and swelling, but there is a difference between an expected effect and an adverse reaction. Make sure your provider shares what is to be expected and what could be *unexpected*—and what can be done to manage it.

How Long It Lasts

Generally, what's great about lasers is that the treatments have a permanent effect on the condition they're treating. They turn back the clock—but your skin continues to age and change as you get older, so new issues will appear.

What Smart Consumers Know

Skin has a huge regenerative capacity, so using resurfacing and exfoliating lasers allows us to get rid of the old and stimulate the new in a way that is very safe, permanent, and cost-effective.

In addition, part of the beauty of these devices is that they might have been devised for cosmetic purposes, but some can also decrease your risk of skin cancer by removing old cells that are potentially precancerous due to chronic radiation damage from decades of sunlight. This is pro-aging: how something you can do to make you look good can also be good for your skin and health.

Lasers are extremely powerful and can be dangerous—they're only as good as the person who has them in hand. Look at them like any musical instrument—clearly, with the same guitar, your average high school musician will play quite differently than Eric Clapton. There is some state variability in who can use these devices, but I firmly believe that only healthcare professionals with appropriate licensure, training, and supervision should prescribe and perform these treatments.

Skin Tightening and Lifting

Radiofrequency and Ultrasound Treatments

Light can only penetrate to certain levels into the skin, so, eventually, we have to harness other sources of energy to target your cosmetic needs. For example, there are lasers that are used to try and melt fat, but the amount of energy required, given the lack of penetration of light to a certain depth, does limit what can be accomplished. This is why other sources of energy have become popular for cosmetic purposes, particularly for their deep skin-tightening benefits. Radiofrequency and ultrasonic wavelengths, like lasers, produce clinically effective heat that falls into this category, using energy from a different place on the electromagnetic spectrum.

Radiofrequency and Ultrasound Work Best For...

These various sources of electromagnetic energies use different techniques to sort of trick the skin to create biological responses that are going to provide rejuvenation. With controlled delivery of this heat up to a particular temperature window, controlled wounds can be created for various purposes. These devices are most commonly used to increase collagen content and improve elasticity for deeper rejuvenation. Thanks to their ability to blindly go through the top layers of the skin, these devices can almost always be used effectively in darker skin tones.

Avoid Them If...

If you expect huge results from just a few visits, avoid these treatments. These devices will not give surgical results.

Pain Scale and Recuperation

Pain can be mild to significant, depending on technology. Bigger per-treatment results come with greater discomfort. Ultrasound treatment, because it can penetrate deeper down into muscle (as seen with technologies such as Ultherapy), can also come with greater discomfort. Mild sedation and analgesia should be offered by your healthcare provider.

When You'll See Results
It often takes a few months to see final differences.

Side Effects
These procedures tend to have the greatest safety profile with relatively no downtime, as they don't affect the upper layers of skin. Mild redness and swelling are extremely temporary, and patients can often return to daily activities immediately.

How Long It Lasts
Generally, the results of therapy are permanent and cumulative, although patients often require and desire maintenance treatments to keep or enhance their effects.

What Smart Consumers Know
Some of the most exciting devices in development are hybrids. For example, one of the hottest technologies now are called energy delivery microneedling devices. Radiofrequency energy is injected and pulsed directly into the depths of the skin, so it doesn't have to be sourced and travel from the outside. These microneedles subsequently give microsecond pulses of heat when they puncture the skin into multiple desired depths, depending on the desired target. Other hybrid devices are combining radiofrequency and laser, radiofrequency and ultrasound, and many other variations.

Volume Optimization

This category covers injectable substances that replace or stimulate lost volume, or that remove fat from certain areas.

The primary treatments are smootheners/fillers, liposuction (physical removal of fat), and various noninvasive devices that destroy fat from the outside, leaving the body to metabolize and excrete it on its own.

Fillers/Smootheners

There are now so many different categories of viscosities and thicknesses for injectables that I actually prefer to use the words "smoothener" and "volumizer" rather than filler—because "filler" is more of a generic word that makes people assume I'm just filling a hole! Whatever the word, smootheners/volumizers are an amazing rejuvenating technique and a safe and easy quick fix when done appropriately. In many instances, these substances can tighten and lift the skin as well. Picture a balloon that has lost air over time. The shape becomes limp and the texture becomes crinkly. By re-volumizing the balloon with air, the shape is lifted and restored, and the quality of the plastic appears to tighten. The art and the success of the end result are in the placement and judgment of where and how much to use.

How They Work

Fillers/Smootheners are substances injected into the skin. They work by hypothetically replacing what has been lost with age. The earliest fillers were made from bovine collagen or were permanent substances like silicone. Now, there is a large range of different types, each with unique properties, some found naturally in our body, and others not. They can be injected in most areas of the face, especially around the mouth, cheeks, and under the eyes, and anywhere else in the body. We even use our own body's fillers to volumize, smoothen, and tighten. For example, for body augmentation and lift, we extract, purify, and inject your body's own fat into the buttock region—sometimes to merely replace lost volume but other times to increase and shape the volume that already exists.

- *Temporary/Reversible.* These are the hyaluronic acid fillers, which are a natural polysaccharide (or sugar) found in skin. They are generally the simplest to use and can be reversed with different levels of ease using an injection of hyaluronidase, an enzyme our body makes. The most popular name brands in the US are Restylane, Juvéderm, Versa, and Belotero. There are several other brands available around the world.

- *Biostimulatory Agents/Semi-Permanent Fillers.* These substances are less about filling or replacing lost volume and more about stimulating your body's own collagen and connective tissue production. They're trickier to use and cannot be readily adjusted or reversed. The most common are calcium hydroxyapatite (Radiesse), and poly-L-lactic acid (Sculptra). They have both short-term and long-term effects and generally last significantly longer than hyaluronic acid fillers.

- *Permanent Fillers.* Decades ago, permanent fillers used to be the only option, but due to complications—if the injections were botched or the body reacted adversely to them, the only option for removal was surgery—they now are used in more limited but essential circumstances. Examples are medical-grade silicone such as Silikon 1000, which I prefer and have extensive experience with as a specialist. Another FDA-approved substance used on- and off-label in the US is Bellafill, made from an artificial agent called polymethyl-methacrylate microspheres (PMMA). Currently, it's only approved for acne scars and, in my opinion and historically, has a higher rate of complication compared to properly used medical-grade silicone oil.

- *Fat Transfer.* With fat transfer, your own fat cells are used, so there is no risk of an allergic reaction. It's best for replacing larger lost volume in the face or body. Treatments are more involved, as they involve harvesting your own fat, and thus can have greater downtime and cost.

Fillers/Smootheners Work Best For...

Fillers work best to create volume, fill lines, smoothen skin, and lift or define tissue on the face or anywhere on the body. They can improve facial smile lines, define jawlines and lips, fill hollow temples, smoothen lip lines, recreate cheekbones giving facial definition, remove dark or hollow eye circles, volumize buttocks, and even improve cellulite.

Avoid Smootheners/Fillers If...

Avoid these if you're not willing to do treatments that require maintenance. You may also want to minimize or avoid them if you have an inherently full or round face. They can create definition, but it may not be worth it to make your face bigger.

How It's Done

Fillers are injected where needed either in one treatment or more slowly over a several-treatment regimen. For fat transfer, your own fat is removed (usually from the buttocks) in a mini-liposuction procedure under local anesthesia and processed so that it can then be re-injected where needed.

Pain Scale and Recuperation

Minimal—recovery is usually minutes to a couple of days, depending on swelling or bruising, mostly. Topical anesthesia is all that is needed in most cases.

When You'll See Results

This is a gratifying procedure as you can see results right away in most circumstances. Depending on the type of filler and the amount, it can take one to two weeks to see the ultimate result. I tell patients not to call me a genius or a quack for at least a week, please! And unless there is something dramatically worrisome, no touch-ups or adjustments until then.

Side Effects

These are often related to the type of filler, the experience of the injector, and the individual patient. Most side effects are generally few and far between, but, sadly, one of the more common is a poor cosmetic outcome requiring fixing. However, the most common and worrisome things to watch for are bruising and swelling from trauma, allergic or hypersensitivity reactions, or accidental injections in or near important blood vessels that could compromise the blood supply to normal tissue. Faulty injections near or compressing blood vessels are rare but certainly can occur. Most of these are all manageable complications that necessitate patients seeking out expert injectors with experience in these situations. Don't forget to ask if your provider has experience in treating potential side effects on any consent form.

How Long It Lasts

This widely depends on the type of filler. It is important to have a conversation with your provider to see what maintenance will be involved to continue the desirable effect. This is of great importance in choosing a filler and has a few variables worth discussing. I tell patients there is no best filler, just as there is no best treatment. Permanent fillers are there for good, unless they are surgically removed, which is why treatments are performed slowly, building over time. Fat transfer is often permanent but can be unpredictable. It's impossible to know how much, if any, your body will harmlessly reabsorb.

I tell patients to unwrap their heads around the "How long does it last?" question. The answer has so many variations and is often based more on the patient than the filler itself. Age, treatment purpose, and physical and genetic factors such as metabolism and lifestyle all affect filler longevity, in addition to how much filler is used. The companies that make these products market them with terminology like "lasts up to six months, one year, two years, etc."—but they take the highest top percentage of patient and filler performance in their studies and then publicize and sell that number. It's deceptive. Have the discussion instead of how often your provider thinks you need to come in to stay looking great. No one wants to wait until the injectables' effect is all gone; it's better to restore the positive effects before the tank is empty, so to speak. I like to "color the roots," to use a hair-coloring metaphor, not reprocess from scratch every time.

> *I tell patients there is no best filler, just as there is no best treatment.*

What Smart Consumers Know

It is essential that consumers seek professional advice from pro-viders who are experienced in the use of several kinds of fillers. Remember my adage: If you only have a hammer, everything looks like a nail. Well, this is especially true here. Start slowly, I always say, as you can always do more. Ask about frequency of maintenance. This will help you budget and understand the maintenance involved.

It is very important to ask your provider if they have ever managed filler complications from the minor to major issues you most definitely should read about before you give consent. If they tell you they have never seen such complications, it clearly means they are not experienced injectors. Complications do rarely occur, and the more you do any activity, the greater the likelihood of seeing and managing problems. This is called experience and expertise.

Most commonly, patients ask, "What if I stop forever—will I be worse off?" The answer is no—all fillers have some degree of biostimulatory effect that helps restore natural tissue, so you will be better off regardless of whether you stop treatment altogether. The only major "worse-off problem" is if you overuse or overfill abusively. This can and will stretch tissue that can ultimately require surgical restoration in the form of a facelift. This again is why too much of a good thing is not always good, and to put yourself in the hands of a provider with enough experience to know the checks and balances of what can be done and overdone. Often, the best injectors say no or enough is enough.

PRP: Platelet-Rich Plasma

PRP has gained a lot of popularity over the years in several fields of medicine. For cosmetic dermatology, your own blood is drawn, and the natural growth factors found in your platelets are isolated via a separation and purification process before being reinjected into your skin. It was originally performed for various orthopedic and joint problems and is now widely used in dermatology, either on its own or in conjunction with other cosmetic techniques, to enhance healing and results. (You may have heard of the "vampire facial" made famous by the Kardashians, who had their own blood rubbed on their faces after a microneedling procedure.)

Although there is little evidence that PRP works for skin rejuvenation, the science shows it is effective for hair growth and wound care. Although there is not enough data to support all of its potential, PRP is being used throughout the body to treat wrinkles, skin quality, cellulite, and dark circles under the eyes, among other cosmetic issues. Ongoing research continues, and I see some but varying degrees of efficacy for various cosmetic concerns. It is not a panacea—it by no means is as effective as pharmaceutical injections or device interventions—but it is worthy of a discussion with your provider whether to use it alone or in conjunction with other treatments.

Fat Removal—Invasive and Noninvasive

Too much in some places and not enough in others—Mother Nature's paradox. Although fat removal is such a broad subject that I could literally write a whole book about it, there are some important facts and myths you need to know when considering fat-removal procedures.

- **Fact #1:** Diet and exercise alone can't always give you the body you desire. We all come in various shapes and sizes, and that's okay. It's also okay to realistically aspire toward the shape you desire. It is your body! People have varying degrees of responsiveness to all efforts in life—don't let this get you down. Take pride in your *pro-activity*! Do not let doctors, personal trainers, nutritionists, life coaches, or anyone else make you feel lazy or a failure if you feel you are honestly putting in the effort and living the pro-aging lifestyle.

- **Fact #2:** Fat removal is *not* a replacement for diet and exercise. These must be maximized before considering fat-removal options. Sadly, even with the greatest of efforts, many people experience unsatisfying irregularities or unevenness in body contours, either from puberty or over time as they age. I always say medical fat removal is for *areas* resistant to diet and exercise, not *people* resistant to diet and exercise.

- **Fact #3:** It is a myth that if you remove fat in one area, it will grow in another. If you keep your weight stable after fat removal, it should stay away. You are born with a fixed number of fat cells. When you gain and lose small amounts of weight, these cells swell and shrink. Only when the body is pushed to significant weight gain do fat cells multiply. So when you destroy or remove fat cells, they should not come back, *but* if you gain a lot of weight, you *will* make more.

- **Fact #4:** The most common question about fat removal is whether to go noninvasive or invasive. A common misconception is that noninvasive is 100 percent safe and without downtime, when that's not necessarily the case.

Noninvasive fat removal is not necessarily better, faster, or safer than liposuction. Noninvasive techniques are generally limited to small amounts of fat removal—teacups relative to soup bowls in the case of liposuction. Although effective, the various noninvasive techniques can have complications and take two to three months to produce any results. Often, more than one treatment may be necessary for desired results, as our bodies can only destroy, metabolize, and excrete small amounts of fat at one time.

- **Fact #5:** Both plastic surgeons and dermatologic surgeons, such as myself, are formally trained to perform liposuction. Most often, plastic surgeons perform traditional liposuction under general anesthesia or IV sedation. Although larger volumes of fat can sometimes be removed in this manner, it is not my opinion that doing so is currently the standard of care. The need to remove more than three liters of fat at a time is usually a sign that patients should lose weight before seeking surgical intervention. With larger amounts removed, there are longer recoveries and higher risk. With the tumescent liposuction I perform, average removal amounts range from half a liter to two and a half liters of pure fat. This is more than enough to make clothing size changes and give the appearance that patients have lost up to ten to fifteen pounds. Traditional liposuction has also proven to be significantly more invasive, with greater risks, longer recovery, and a higher rate of poor cosmetic outcomes due to skin irregularities caused by larger instrumentation.

Tumescent liposuction performed under local anesthesia remains the safest, most predictable option, and offers the most cosmetically appealing and permanent body sculpting to date. It is more of a meticulous sculpting procedure that takes more time and finesse but is well worth it. It remains today the most satisfying, predictable, and safest procedure I perform for both myself and my patients.

Invasive Fat Removal: Tumescent Liposuction

Liposuction Works Best For...

I always tell people, "Come to me for the *last* five to ten pounds, not the *first* five to ten." Liposuction targets specific areas of intractable fat, like love handles, a belly, thighs, or anywhere unwanted fat exists above the muscle and below the skin. It works on *cosmetic* fat, meaning pinchable, grab-able fat, not visceral fat, which is found under the muscle and surrounds the organs (this is what makes body parts merely look distended or thick).

> *"Come to me for the* last *five to ten pounds, not the* first *five to ten."*

As you read already, it's not meant for anyone who has eating or obesity problems—it's for those that exercise regularly and eat a healthy diet, or perhaps can't lose those last few pounds.

Avoid Liposuction If...

If liposuction is sold to you as a weight-loss technique, you will be wasting your time, energy, and money. You actually don't lose as many pounds as you *look* like you do. I may be able to make someone look like they lost ten pounds in the right place, but they may only notice a two-pound difference on the scale. Actual weight loss is clearly more than fat reduction.

How It's Done

Liposuction used to be more commonly done under general anesthesia, which made it much more difficult, traumatic, riskier, and expensive for patients. Now the technique of performing it under local anesthesia is the standard. Invented, advanced, and popularized by a small group of dermatologic surgeons in the 1980s and 1990s, including my mentor, Dr. Rhoda Narins, tumescent liposuction injects patients with large volumes of a very low-dose Lidocaine solution into the targeted areas. Like going to the dentist, this is the only part that is felt at all by the patient. Mild to moderate conscious sedation is often offered. Patients can even go to the bathroom during this procedure. Once the patient is numb and comfortable, a series of micro-cannulas of varying shapes and sizes slowly sculpt out the fat by hand and motorized suction. Think playing a violin rather than jackhammering—this is a sculpting process. Sometimes I use technologies to melt the fat first or help tighten the skin from the inside, but for all intents and purposes, the procedure hasn't changed much since my training. And, in my opinion, it is the biggest contribution to aesthetic medicine that dermatologists have made historically. The diluted form of anesthesia that was developed during the discovery of this technique is used throughout medicine for various purposes to provide safe surgery without the need for general anesthesia.

Pain Scale and Recuperation

There is very little to no pain with this technique. Certainly, none that requires prescription pain relief after the procedure. When the local anesthesia wears off, you will feel soreness, at most. Most people need only a twenty-four- to forty-eight-hour recovery. They can go back to work in two days and can be back in the gym in one week. For most patients, a Spanx-like compression garment is worn under clothing for about a week, which helps healing and prevents complications, but recovery is quick. After doing over five thousand treatments in twenty years, I have yet to see a single significant medical complication.

When You'll See Results

Patients often see some results the next day, and overwhelming changes within a month. Ultimate skin-tightening results are seen in four to six months.

Side Effects

Regardless of its safety, tumescent liposuction is still a surgical procedure, even if it is a minimally invasive one. One that requires skill, experience, art, and surgical precautions as does any other surgical procedure. Results are predictable, and it is extremely safe when performed by the right hands. Mild to moderate bruising and swelling can be expected. Infections and skin irregularities are what to watch out for and are most commonly preventable and treatable.

How Long It Lasts

Liposuction lasts as long as your weight remains the same or goes down. If you take fat out and then gain twenty pounds, the new fat has to go somewhere—not where you took out the fat cells, but you still have fat cells everywhere else in your body, and they're going to grow when you gain weight. So the first question I always ask a potential liposuction candidate is if their weight has changed in the last year. If it's gone down, liposuction might be an option. If it's gone up, they need to consider managing that before undergoing the procedure.

What Smart Consumers Know

The paradox of liposuction is that I don't make fat people skinny; I just make people more symmetrical. No matter how much weight some people lose, their bottom looks completely different than their top. Or some people are rail-thin, yet they have their father's arms and mother's neck or chest that are disproportionate to the rest of their body.

Liposuction is an option for those who were told by their doctors to lose thirty pounds, worked really hard to lose twenty pounds, and then couldn't get the scale to budge, no matter what. There's nothing worse than when you're doing better for yourself and you don't see results! For them, liposuction is that extra little push. It not only makes them feel better about the now, but it also empowers them to move forward. This is pro-aging in action: Any kind of self-care you do to look better makes you want to do it more. It's auto-contagious positivity!

Noninvasive Fat Removal

There are several noninvasive fat-removal options on the market. All rely on a similar principle to target fat from the outside of the skin, causing inflammation and destruction of fat cells, and subsequent metabolism and excretion from the body. CoolSculpting is probably the most popularly performed as it was the first major player in the arena. Other devices, such as SculpSure (which uses laser heat), UltraShape (ultrasound energy) Vanquish and truSculpt (radiofrequency), and various other crossover devices such as Emsculpt (magnetic field technology) now add a broad spectrum of options. Again, there is no best. Each device has its own pros and cons. I use many of them in my practice, some more often than others.

How CoolSculpting and Other Devices Work

CoolSculpting, or fat freezing, relies on a biological phenomenon that, by reducing the temperature of skin to a certain freezing point, the fat cells go through apoptosis, akin to an auto-destruct mechanism, without damaging the outside layers of the skin. A certain degree of fat can be removed with this technique, dependent on the size and shape of the applicator, as your body can dissolve and metabolize the fat on its own. Other devices mentioned above cause similar types of inflammation and metabolism to remove fat in the same way.

Noninvasive Fat Removal Works Best For...

This is ideal for someone who has three to five pounds to lose in generally localized areas. Larger areas can be addressed with multiple cycles of treatments and overlapping of treatment zones and handpieces. They may be ideal for patients who, for medical reasons, cannot get liposuction. For larger areas, though, tumescent liposuction is generally a better option.

Avoid Noninvasive Fat Removal If...

This isn't the treatment for you if you're looking for overall weight reduction or wanting to dramatically alter body shape.

How It's Done

Most treatments are performed by attaching a treatment handpiece to the targeted areas. Different technologies have handpieces with different shapes and ergonomic variations that may make them better for some patients than others. Treatment times usually vary from twenty minutes to an hour. Most patients can immediately resume their daily activities after treatment.

Pain Scale and Recuperation

These treatments are not painless and without recovery. Treatment areas can be bruised, inflamed, sore, hypersensitive, or even numb for days to weeks. No matter which way you cut the cake, the destruction of fat causes inflammation, and inflammation requires recovery.

When You'll See Results

It takes much longer than liposuction to see results—usually a minimum of eight to twelve weeks. You must also wait this amount of time between treatments to minimize complications. This can be frustrating for patients.

Side Effects

There can be long-term numbing, bruising, burns, and irregularities in the skin afterward due to unevenness of the fat removal. These machines should never just be attached to the patient and switched on.

How Long It Lasts

As with liposuction, if your weight remains the same, the effects are permanent.

What Smart Consumers Know

As with anything in cosmetic dermatology, there's no best noninvasive fat-removal device. There is something out there for everybody, however. I have most of the devices and have used them in different instances. But I always tell my patients that you can only burn so much garbage in your backyard before it has to be carted out. So the most important factor is candidate selection.

The effects from all noninvasive fat-removal devices are limited. You can only remove a small amount at a time, and it often requires several treatments in several areas. You just can't do the whole belly or the whole midsection or the lower section of the body. For some patients, I'll recommend liposuction for certain areas and one of several noninvasive devices for others. You have to find the right way to get the ball into the hole there!

Most important is for you to be offered the full spectrum of available devices. Unfortunately, a huge number of med spas throughout the country do not offer any form of liposuction, and they only have one type of noninvasive device. Of course, you're only going to get one procedure sold to you if you go to a place like that.

You also need to have all the short-term and long-term risks, the course of recovery, and the number of treatments explained to you for informed consent. For many patients, the most cost-effective, time-effective, least-traumatic, safest, and best cosmetic results will be with tumescent liposuction. Understandably, some people will not want even minor surgery performed, despite the fact that any scarring is usually negligible and there is minimal risk or trauma.

Muscle-Development Technologies

Originally created by a company that has a patent on what's called HIFEM (high-intensity focused electromagnetic) technology, Emsculpt is the hottest device in my office right now. Many companies are currently in the race to develop competing technologies and advance the realm of this exciting field of rejuvenation.

How Emsculpt Works

It uses a focused magnetic field to hyperstimulate the motor neurons of a muscle group. It challenges the muscle in a way that you can't do voluntarily—when you're exercising, you're flexing 40–60 percent of that muscle group every three to five seconds. This machine contracts 100 percent of the muscle, *twenty thousand times* in a thirty-minute period, without recruiting or causing strain on all of the other muscles in your body.

Emsculpt Works Best For...
I use it on the belly, buttocks, arms, and legs, for more muscle definition and bulk. It can also be used on those who've had muscle issues and are recovering from surgery or injury; it can dramatically speed up recuperation. Research is currently being done to assess its benefits for general core development and well-being.

Avoid Emsculpt If...
If you have any non-titanium metal or battery-operated electronic parts in your body, avoid Emsculpt. But if you can have an MRI, you can get this done.

How It's Done
Panels are placed on the area to be treated, and the intensity is gradually increased during the course of the treatment, much like the slow increase in intensity of any workout plan. Four approximately thirty-minute treatments are performed in a two-week period.

Pain Scale and Recuperation
The treated area might be sore for a few hours or a day, in a similar manner to an intense workout. You should not be in pain during treatment. You may feel strain on the muscle, but it should be controlled by your feedback and the performance of your healthcare provider—your "Emsculpt trainer."

When You'll See Results
As with exercise, muscle swelling is also seen immediately with this technology. Longer-term and permanent results are seen over weeks to months.

Side Effects

Emsculpt can cause muscle strain and, like any medical device, must be performed on patients by a trained healthcare professional. It is not a toy, nor should it be found in health clubs—only in doctors' offices. You can get hurt using this technology.

How Long It Lasts

As with many other treatments, this varies considerably. It's like asking how long the benefits of a monthlong series of daily spin classes last. What is apparent from clinical studies is that long-lasting biologic changes occur in the redevelopment of muscle tissue, and the effects are such that they can't be duplicated with exercise alone. This technology is not a cheat—it's a magnifier to exercise and the lifestyle of maintaining strength.

What Smart Consumers Know

As we get older, one of the major limitations we have is the ability to exercise and get the type of muscle development that we want without injury. Older muscles are replaced by fat, but if you build up the muscle again, it destroys the local fat cells. You can't remove belly fat with sit-ups, but you can with Emsculpt. This device is now doing for the muscle-development market what Botox did for the wrinkle-reduction market at the turn of the millennium. It helps you regain muscle strength in a way that's impossible for you to do on your own.

When I first starting using this machine, I was amazed. I have two of them and am investing in a third machine. I once again had that aha moment of seeing the forest through the trees, as I did when I first tried Botox in my forehead. I originally thought Emsculpt would work best for those who were already in great shape and just wanted an extra pack in their six-pack. Fortunately, we're learning that people of all shapes and sizes are getting an enormous sense of wellness and postural improvement when they use Emsculpt on their belly area, thanks to how efficiently it works the core muscles. It's not a replacement for a healthy diet or regular aerobic exercise, but it is an excellent complement and, when performed appropriately, should not cause any injuries as exercising can. Patients who were slightly overweight and seemingly not ideal candidates are thrilled with the results and tell me they stand and walk straighter, have less back pain, and can do yoga and other exercises better. They're more confident and more motivated, and that, of course, makes them more beautiful.

Cosmetic Dermatology vs. Plastic Surgery

When I was doing my medical training in the 1990s, plastic surgeons concentrated on surgical procedures. They considered themselves "real" surgeons—not "just" doctors who messed around with collagen injections and chemical peels.

How things have changed! Many plastic surgeons are now doing the same kind of treatments that I do—but cosmetic dermatologists generally don't do the level of invasive surgeries plastic surgeons perform. Thanks to technological advances with devices and drugs, there are now many more options for a spectrum of results. You might be able to have injectables and lasers make you look more youthful or vibrant as an alternative to a facelift. In my opinion, the need for plastic surgery isn't going anywhere. In fact, these dermatologic procedures are, I believe, a gateway for patients to feel more comfortable about eventual surgical intervention. Again, pro-aging is about sourcing available options and combining what's right for you.

At some point, though, the law of diminishing returns kicks in.

Some people do not want surgery under any circumstances, as they fear the anesthesia, pain, risk, or they don't have time to take off for the recuperation period. Or, understandably, they are wary and don't think it's worth the trouble. Some people will always opt for surgery as their first choice as the effects are long-lasting and they just want to get it over with. Some people will stop having any treatments, surgical or nonsurgical. This is an informed decision only you can make.

Most important to understand is that surgery is not necessarily a replacement for cosmetic dermatology but a complement to it. Patients often come back months later for lasers and injectables, but certainly the approach and amounts may differ. For example, a facelift does little for wrinkles around the mouth or in between the eyes, or to fix sun damage. Fillers, neuromodulators, and lasers still need to be done to address different concerns.

To help you make the best possible choices, I spoke with my dear friend and world-renowned colleague Dr. David Rosenberg, who is board-certified in both facial plastic surgery and otolaryngology-head and neck surgery, about these issues.

Thinking About Plastic Surgery

A Q&A with Dr. David Rosenberg, a leading facial plastic surgeon known for creating the most natural results with the shortest recovery time possible.

Do cosmetic dermatologists downplay the need for surgery and plastic surgeons downplay what noninvasive cosmetic procedures can do?

When a facial plastic surgeon is very busy and operating at maximum capacity, they're not going to be speaking out of a need for added income—they're going to be speaking out of concern for the best interest of the patient. In my practice, I do not perform injectables. I refer these patients to others. When a person doesn't need to count every dollar, there is a role for surgery and there is a continued role for nonsurgical interventions. In my mind, the best people to perform injectables and the nonsurgical intervention are the skin experts, the dermatologists. The best person to perform invasive surgery is a facial plastic surgeon.

When do you know it's time to move on from less-invasive procedures to more invasive surgery?

Part of it is driven by the patient's desire, and part of it is going to be determined by the dermatologist guiding the patient. The patient absolutely has to be intimately involved in the decision process.

One scenario is that certain patients will be of the mindset that they don't want to keep getting injectables that require them to see the doctor every four to six months. Injectables are not without recovery time, so if the patient has surgery, they'll have much less need for fillers. This typically happens when people are in their early fifties and are seeing jowls and a loose neck, and the patients just want to move on so they don't have to think about it.

The other scenario is patients who want to do nonsurgical treatments for as long as possible but, at a certain point, will reach the limit of benefits provided. We've all seen instances where dermatologists are adding so much volume with filler that the jowls might seem diminished, but the volume of the face has become distorted. It's become rounder. The unique architecture of the face has changed. When these people smile, there are two apples on each side that expand the size of their face, so they end up looking as fake as if they'd had a bad facelift.

Is a facelift a replacement for less invasive dermatology procedures or more of a complement?

It's both. When a facelift is well done, it diminishes the need for filler in the cheeks by a large degree because I'm lifting the cheek pad onto the cheekbone again.

There are things a facelift can't do:

- It's not a replacement for filler in the marionette lines or the downturn of the corners of the mouth; those are improved with a facelift but not eliminated. For those issues, filler is extremely advisable, and patient communication is essential so they understand why. They would need less filler than before but still have it for maintenance.

- Excessive heaviness of the brows can only be treated with an endoscopic brow lift. Glabellar lines (frown lines) are the result of expression, and you're still going to have expression because those muscles underneath are still working. Botox and other neuromodulators can temporarily raise the brows, mostly in people under the age of fifty, but they become less effective over the years. There comes a point when you can't treat forehead lines with neuromodulators at all if you are trying to achieve maximum lift of the brows—thus the need for surgical intervention. For better or worse, glabellar lines and crow's-feet can only be treated with neuromodulators, so Botox will absolutely be needed afterward to maintain the degree of smoothness the patient is pursuing.

What's the most important thing to know before going into a plastic surgery consult?

I think that every person should walk into the exam room having looked at the doctor's web page and assessed it critically. Is the web page there to inform the patient? Or is it there to achieve maximum search-engine optimization and get more patients? Look at every result and ask yourself if these are appropriate results for your goals. Take a realistic look at the reviews. Do they seem authentic, or are they plugs? When you arrive at the office, is it welcoming or not welcoming? Is the office clean? Is the staff supportive? Details. I always tell my patients to look at these areas and compare them to the next office. Ultimately, it's about rapport with the surgeon and the feeling that they will meet your needs and expectations. The surgery itself is only part of the care. The pre-op, the post-op, and the nursing care are all very important in getting the safest and best results. Certainly, word-of-mouth recommendations are very useful in picking a surgeon of any kind as well.

How have the aesthetics of plastic surgery changed?

When I started my practice in 2000, the most prolific surgeons in the New York region were famous for creating the tightest necks and tightest faces out there. Whoever could create that tight look was considered the most talented. I looked at those results and did not see beauty—I saw evidence of surgery and a severity of look that was not natural. What I perceived as an undesirable result was an assessment of what I saw performed. That made me an outlier. At the same time, an operation called a deep-plane facelift was gaining some popularity, and the benefit was that it allowed for a rejuvenation that wasn't evident to the casual observer. A person could look beautiful and celebrate their appearance without looking like work had been done. That's been the major shift from 2000 to now—it's the essence of the maturity and sophistication of aesthetic work. Looking like yourself is the most beautiful. The word "tight" is not an appropriate goal. A face is never tight; it's contoured and defined, but tight is an artificiality. I want my patients to appear *authentic*. I want them to look like themselves. And what makes people who come to me unhappy with their looks is that they have jowls and a loose neck or bags under their eyes. It's not that they're fifty-eight years old that bothers them as much as that they look worn, yet they feel fit. How they feel internally is at odds with how they look externally. That is where I bring my patients into balance. I never hear my patients say, "Make me look fifteen years younger." They say, "Make me look great now." It's a very different goal. I want to make my patients look as beautiful as possible as quickly as possible with the longest duration of benefits.

It's what you call pro-aging!

Let's Talk About Teeth

Your smile and the health of your teeth are incredibly important components of pro-aging. Teeth that are neglected are not only a health risk, but they instantly age your appearance. I spoke to Dr. Michael Apa—one of the world's most renowned aesthetic dentists and a close colleague with whom I share many patients—to get his views about how your teeth and smile not only affect the way you look but the way you live.

Thinking About a Better Smile

Q&A with Dr. Michael Apa, celebrity cosmetic dentist and founder of Apa Aesthetic.

What is the difference between cosmetic dentistry and aesthetic dentistry?

One of the first things you have to do is define cosmetic dentistry. Cosmetic dentistry is like press-on fake nails, treating only the surface appearance of the teeth. Aesthetic dentistry is full, functional, rehabilitation dentistry with an accent on results looking correct. They are very different types of dentistry.

How do your teeth affect how you age?

When we talk about pro-aging, you have to think about your teeth as the foundation of your face. They're the structure that supports the lower third of your face. If you see someone who has dentures and takes them out, their whole face collapses; when they put the dentures back in, their face fills out again.

Your teeth are controlled by your muscles. People also have a side they favor when they grind their teeth. Left, right, or front. As a result, they'll have one really full cheek and one really angular cheek, and that will start to pull the bone. Why do you think people become asymmetrical over time? Their face structure changes shape. The bones move, pulled by muscle. The fat and the collagen and elastin change. What people don't understand is that your chin shifts, and one side becomes full and strong and the other side becomes weak. And then there's stress and external factors that can wear on the structure of the mouth—grinding, gum recession, changes in your bite, among others.

So, since I'm not performing dermatology or plastic surgery and I'm asked what the order is that you should prioritize your anti-aging treatments, teeth should be first. Of course, it's a health thing. But even one step further is how you look at someone's face. With a facelift, you're tightening to a level where the patient looks youthful again. If you tighten someone's face who took out their dentures, versus tightening the face of someone who put those dentures back in, you'd do much less tightening or filling because you'd have much less volume there.

What I'm saying is, with dentistry, you're reconstructing the foundation of the house. The siding and the windows and the roof and all of those things are the skin. Once you set the foundation, there's less to do in terms of how teeth affect lip support or cheek volume. In other words, you could hypothetically need less filler if you treated your teeth properly. Especially as people lose teeth as they get older, and this affects the symmetry of their face. Of course, none of us are trying to create complete symmetry, because that doesn't exist. We're simply trying to create harmony in each individual patient's face.

What can you do in terms of being proactive in staving off the natural aging process of your teeth as you get older?

The number-one thing is, if you wore braces, that pretty much sets your structure up and then you should retain that position with bonded wires, which are permanent retainers. That will save you so much time in the future. If you can't afford an aesthetic dentist, the next best thing is using a custom-fit night guard, which will save you a lot of bone and gum loss.

As for OTC whitening, you have to set your expectations. You see a Crest commercial and it shows you perfectly white teeth, but whitening kits can only give you a slightly whiter version of your teeth as they are now. And, actually, very few people can benefit the way you think from whitening. First of all, your tooth structure has to be there. You can't have worn or chipped teeth, old crowns, or fillings in the front of your mouth, as they won't bleach. The other thing is, whitening makes teeth *brighter*, not whiter. It reflects more light off your teeth; it's not actually changing the color—it's changing the perception. Plus, it only lasts for a month, and professional whitening doesn't last much longer.

What can aesthetic dentistry do to enhance your appearance, especially as you're getting older?

Some patients come in and think they want straight, white teeth; they're thinking cosmetic. Other patients come in and say, "I don't want straight, white teeth—I want my bite fixed." They're thinking functional. But the truth is they're the same people. As a good dentist, you want to meet your patients' expectations in a realistic manner, while making them look and feel better.

As we age, the upper lip gets longer and thinner, so it can give volume back to your upper lip. You lose cheek fat, which everyone's trying to fill. Aesthetic dentistry will make your cheeks and face look fuller without putting any filler in them. It also changes your skin tone. If your skin is fair and your teeth are dark, it draws the color out of your skin. Whiter teeth on a fair person can essentially change the perception of their skin tone, which makes them look healthier. When your teeth don't look good and you put all that back to where it should be, you're immediately going to look healthier.

The interesting thing about teeth is that they're the silent secret weapon of people's confidence. If I have a gigantic pimple or a cold sore on my face, I won't be interacting or talking to people in the same way I would if my skin were clear. People have the same insecurity about teeth. I can change this after just three hours in my chair. You don't have to go on a diet for two years. After I fix their teeth, I see my patients six months later and their hair is different, they've lost five pounds, and they're dressing better. They're carrying themselves completely differently because their not wanting to open their mouths had been holding them back. I see that all the time, and it's very special.

Why are teeth so neglected as we get older?

In this country, unfortunately, good dentistry, whether aesthetic or not, is very expensive. A dermatologist can put filler in your cheeks or your upper lip and you'll be happy, and it's much more accessible to many more people because it's affordable in the short term. You can't do just one tooth in my type of dentistry. It needs continual upkeep, and it has to be replaced after fifteen years. So not many people are talking about it, and not many doctors are trained in it.

What happens is that people don't prioritize taking care of themselves, let alone the contents of their mouth. Their teeth always fall last on the list because they think nobody needs to see them. But it's never too late to start taking care of them.

Phew! This chapter is full of a lot info, right? I did my best to concisely review the technologies, the tricks, and the approaches for modern-day cosmetic enhancement. Clearly, I left out many details. The point is not to overwhelm you with endless information—you are getting enough of that in every aspect of the world today. It can be confusing, but it is, at the very least, extremely exciting. The world of aesthetic medicine is growing exponentially, and so are safe options to balance what we see in the mirror and what we feel inside.

I am often asked, "Doc, when do I just give up the fight and let it all go? When is it not worth it anymore?" My answer is always the same: If you feel good, then why wouldn't you want to look like the best version of yourself? What we face every single day is our own image reflected back to us. We deserve to feel good about that if we have the health and the means.

> *"When is it not worth it anymore?" My answer is always the same: If you feel good, then why wouldn't you want to look like the best version of yourself?*

CHAPTER 5

Connect with Community

There are no bad pictures; that's just how your face
looks sometimes.

—ABRAHAM LINCOLN

I always thought I would become a psychologist or a psychiatrist. I was a neuro-psych major at Vassar, a very liberal arts school that, when I attended, had far more female than male students, so it was wonderfully feminine and artistic and creative. It was where, I realized years later, I learned more about becoming a cosmetic dermatologist than I did in medical school or residency. My female friends, professors, classmates, and the overall empathetic environment taught me so much about people, not just women, but also the varying themes of gender, sexual preference, beauty, art, political and social diversity...all while I was concurrently studying science and going pre-med. These influences all seems quite commonplace now, but in the mid-1980s, we were living during the AIDS crisis and the conservative excess of the period. Needless to say, many universities and their student bodies at this time were not as open-minded.

So much of who I am today was rooted in this period and the preceding years spent with my peers at The Horace Mann School in the Bronx; I'm still very close with many of them, thirty-five years later. They later laughed with me when I joked about switching from psychiatry to dermatology because, I told them, Botox worked better than Prozac to make you feel better about yourself. Every day of my life, I use my psychology training and value many of my skills as a function of learning and dealing with people in regard to their thoughts about themselves.

My classmates and academic experiences also taught me the true meaning of community, which has extended to every aspect of my practice—and how I live.

Building Your Community Is Always Based on Trust (Just Like with Your Providers!)

My patients have all become part of the PFRANKMD community, and they *are* the most important part of my work. Because my treatments with them are so professionally intimate, I hear about their relationships, their illnesses, their struggles with themselves, their struggles at work, the good times and bad times. I rejoice with them when they tell me about the bar mitzvahs and christenings and weddings. And then I tease them that I hope I get photo credit in the party pictures!

What are we really discussing when we share information about our lives? *Community.* And how being part of a community is an essential part of pro-aging. Because the people and the energy we surround ourselves with have such a direct impact on our own self-perception.

With all our concerns, both physical and mental, we are all special *but not* uncommon. *We're all aging, and understandably, we all want to do something about it!*

One conversation that links many of my patients to my community is the one where I assure them that with all our concerns, both physical and mental, we are all *special* but not *uncommon*. We're all aging, and understandably, we all want to do something about it! Almost everyone who sits down for their first consultation thinks that they're the first and only person on this planet with that specific issue. (This is also true whether you're going to a psychiatrist, a nutritionist, a personal trainer, or your child's teacher for that first parent-teacher conference.) Because that's what we do: We put ourselves in a corner. We put ourselves in a corner when we raise children, and when we're struggling with work and relationships and tell ourselves that no one else can possibly understand just how bad we feel. "My situation may be similar, but this is different," we say to ourselves.

We especially put ourselves in the corner when dealing with physical self-image and how we feel when we look in the mirror every day. I've had enough experience with a variety of issues so that I can give each patient the options they're looking for. Everyone's a little different. Everybody is special. I'm not going to treat you the same as I do everybody else. My work is not one size fits all. I'm not going to do the filler in the same way that I'm going to do for my next patient. Our paths don't have to be the same nor do we have to feel like we are either giving in or giving up.

One of the greatest gifts of my practice and my teaching is that I've been able to surround myself with people who are receptive to my help and in return are additional sorts of inspiration to my business and my life. We give each other much-needed perspective. Any business, whether it's Apple, Amazon, the deli on the corner, or a dermatologist, will be successful only when it strives to connect with its audience, taking in both good and bad feedback and striving to constantly improve those connections.

The most important gauge for happiness is your relationships within your community—with your friends, family, colleagues—all the people you're intimate with. Communities can have negative aspects too, of course. There have been countless psychological studies about social pressure, not just in the way you look, but in the way you act and what people do alone in a room, versus when others are there. Some people have negative social pressures at school and at work, with their families or their religion, that they find to be inescapable or harmful. That's when a healthy dose of pro-aging self-love is most needed to help you do what's best for *you*.

This is why the community aspect is such an important part of the pro-aging philosophy. We are all connected. You with yourself and your loved ones and colleagues. You with the world.

> *We are all connected. You with yourself and your loved ones and colleagues. You with the world.*

And, of course, when do people feel the most beautiful? When they connect with another human being in real life, not online. No one shines more or looks better than when they're in love, as I'm sure you know. Those who isolate themselves from live personal contact cannot look beautiful because they don't *feel* beautiful.

Self-Image and Finding Your Place in Your Community

One of the ways we as people connect with each other is through shared experiences, especially about our appearance. My patients quickly come to learn that they can confide in me about their insecurities, especially when I share stories about my own physical and popularity deficits as a pre-teen. I was chubby and physically awkward—athletics were not a part of my early childhood. Even after I slimmed down and became fit, at Vassar College and even up until med school I still had a lot of trepidation and insecurities because, as a student at an extremely competitive high school, I felt that everyone else there was smarter than me. I'd always been told that I had a lot of potential but that I couldn't focus. I fell into the trap where my perception fed my destiny.

Fortunately, only with time did I learn otherwise. And I also had an amazing shift in my self-image due to something no one believes when I first tell them: I was a roller disco diva!

The Roller-Disco Community Changed My Life

As I mentioned, my father was a dentist (and is still practicing at the age of seventy-eight!) and my mother was a nurse, but they both loved music and dancing and decided to take a break from dealing with teeth and patients all day. They opened two roller skating rinks in Brooklyn, so, while all of my friends were going to camp or playing on sports teams or just hanging out, I spent every weekend of my pre-teen years in the rink, dancing with the regulars. That's what deepened my love and appreciation for music, and that's what changed my body from a husky kid to a more physically and emotionally secure teenager. It gave me more confidence, rhythm, physical strength, and swagger.

It also gave me access to an entirely different community of people who came together through their love of roller skating. Our discos were in Bedford-Stuyvesant and Fort Greene, near where my father's practice was located. These areas are now filled with million-dollar condos, but, back then, they were underprivileged and rough neighborhoods where few white, middle-class families like my own lived. They loved my dad, the roller-disco dentist, and we loved the environment that they all lit up. They were part of my *community* during these important formative years.

Spending every weekend in the roller disco for over four years was the landmark period of my young life. I was integrally involved, and I slept in the back during the all-night 7 p.m. to 7 a.m. skate sessions on Saturday nights. I saw how the skaters used their skate time to mitigate their stress. I was surrounded by a lot of people who had a lot less than me yet in many ways were as happy as many of my classmates and friends who from the outside had so much more.

For better or worse, I learned early on that the way you look is not your most important quality but is still an integral part of your self-image. Roller skating transformed me physically—I didn't start skating with the thought that I'd lose weight and get buff; it just happened because it's incredibly good exercise and was so much fun that I'd be on my skates for hours. The more I slimmed down and shaped up, the more I was treated differently. The people who may have teased me a bit and the classmates, who had ignored me when I was speaking in class, suddenly wanted to hang out with me. Other kids started paying more attention to me too.

That's when I started to learn an incredibly valuable life lesson. Everyone always says, "Just be yourself and you'll be fine." But that was *wrong*. I was *myself* when I was eleven and being ignored every day, and I was still being *myself* three years later when everyone wanted to be my friend. Because there is no one self. The self is always mutable as it accumulates experience and, hopefully, wisdom and guidance as you surround yourself with the things that will mold you into the person that is "yourself." Yes, we all have certain personality traits, but an eighteen-year-old who's taken out of rural Iowa to go fight in Afghanistan has become a different self when he returns from war. So I was a little bit resentful of this shift in my friends' attitude at first—asking myself why they hadn't liked me when I felt like I was still the same person inside as I'd been when I was *chubby*—but then I started to take advantage of it, I'm sorry to say. It took me more than another decade to find that balance and stop letting insecurities drive my demeanor and actions.

The transformation from all that awkwardness and discontent taught me to be positive through the power of aesthetic influence.

I realized what the power of physical attractiveness was and what it attracted. But I only appreciated it because I hadn't had it before.

And I appreciated it the most because my community—the community of roller disco skaters in deepest Brooklyn—had never once judged me. They didn't care if I was pudgy and gawky or slim and sleek, rich or poor. I was there, dancing, and sharing an endorphin high with others who felt exactly the same way! I felt good about myself for the first time.

The roller disco also helped shape me as an eclectic adult. Artistically, creatively, and professionally, there's no point in being "normal" if you truly want to succeed. It's not so much a matter of being *better*; it's a matter of being *different* and wanting to stand out. It makes me want to try new techniques and devices all the time and look at my work and my business from a different perspective, because there's no point in being like every other cosmetic dermatologist. I always wanted to be different, once I realized the power it could harness. And I realized that you shouldn't ever feel guilty about wanting to be unique, just as you shouldn't ever about feel guilty about wanting to look better. That's the essence of the pro-aging philosophy!

I still have my old roller skates with the custom lights on the wheels as they spin and, for the first time in over decade, I put them on recently (they actually still fit!). My wife did not appreciate the scuffed-up floors in our living room. Crank up the music and I can still make the magic on eight wheels. It is as ingrained in me as riding a bike, and nothing gives me more of a rush.

The Fitness Community Can Change Your Life Too

The positive social "pressure" of working out with a group of people can change your life too. Believe me: If we didn't have positive social pressures, we'd be running around like the young boys in *Lord of the Flies*!

The internet has totally transformed the ability to work out if you can't get to classes in a gym or studio. All you have to do is turn on your computer or TV and be instantly connected to a virtual community of people from all over the world. You can exercise to a prerecorded class or many other workout-type sessions, interacting with a live class.

I've had hundreds of patients tell me over the years how they hated working out until they found a class they loved. For them, it's not just about getting stronger and more fit. It's about the camaraderie of shared goals and the motivation and encouragement they give each other. We're social creatures, after all, and what could be more fun than learning how to dance or box or do martial arts or just go for a brisk walk with a group? It makes you feel good in every possible way. Social pressure is not always a bad thing. It can give us great strength and motivation and subsequently amazing results in our life. The real trick is to choose the right influences, influencers, and to surround yourself with the community of social pressures that will suit your desired goals.

The Pros and Cons of Social Media

As you've learned already, looking your very best and doing things for or to your body must be because you want to do them for yourself, never for somebody else. You have to be good enough for yourself first. Not because someone in your office made a crack about your laugh lines or because you're going through a painful breakup. This is where cosmetic rejuvenation, social intimacy, and social media are all folded into each other.

You have to be good enough for yourself first.

The Positive Aspects of Social Media

Social media has utterly changed how we see the world and ourselves. There's so much good to be found thanks to our online world. With just the hit of a few keys, we can instantly search for even the most arcane bits of information and discover encyclopedias' worth of knowledge. We have access to professional associations and medical sites that provide vetted, authoritative information about any and every condition. There are countless links to news sites and commentary about anything you could imagine, in every country of the world.

I was hesitant about social media and actually poo-pooed it a couple of years ago. I'm glad now that I changed my mind and set up my feed on Instagram, as it's been nothing but positive in terms of the education I can provide and the feedback I get. It's become an excellent way for people to learn about me and my work and for me to be able to project the personality of my practice. Through trial and error, I've learned what I can and cannot share, what works and what doesn't. As with anything else, it's all about *authenticity*.

I have learned that when you deliver your version of authenticity to any pursuit or endeavor, you have the greatest chance of achieving personal and professional success. Trying to be like someone other than yourself solely on the exterior, rather than through personal growth, only leads to a dead end. It is therefore essential to always recognize the balance between your persona and your person when interacting with the manipulative nature of the online world. This is true whether you're on an online dating site or running a billion-dollar business.

And, of course, cosmetic healthcare practitioners have websites that are full of helpful tips. You can see the options offered by a particular provider, which can help streamline your search. You can get an idea of their aesthetic and philosophy.

Just as important is that social media has created a virtual community that has connected people in ways we never could have dreamed of before we were able to go online. Being able to talk to anyone for free practically anywhere in the world in an amazing gift. Online support groups can be literal lifesavers and give you reams of information and advice you wouldn't have access to otherwise. Sites like Facebook, Instagram, and Twitter can connect you with like-minded friends and keep you on the pulse of what's going on every sphere of life.

The Negative Aspects of Social Media and Selfie Culture: How the Fake World Affects Your Psyche and Makes It Harder to Connect

I wish I didn't see so many patients come to me solely due to the pressures of social media for photos—moms who want a cosmetic treatment for the first time only because their child is getting married, not because it's something they really want, for example. Budgets for weddings used to be about the caterers and the ice sculptures. Now you have to factor in mom's laser treatments and liposuction. All of this is okay, as long as it's for the right reasons.

Dr. Michael Apa and I often discuss how smiling is the most important form of live communication and is a predictor for well-being, happiness, and beauty. Smiling starts when we're babies, copying the funny faces our thrilled parents are making at us to try and communicate how happy they are to have us in their lives. You can't fake it and you can't inject a smile—and its greatest impact is always *in person*.

The Selfie Generation

Don't get me started on filters and other modification apps. Selfies and cellphone photos have created a huge culture of photo modification to undo the damage done by cellphone lenses and life.

They can make you look great on your phone—erasing lines and wrinkles and jowls, improving skin tone, making acne and scars disappear.

So, as much as people love taking photos of themselves, *looking* objectively at those photos has become very difficult. As a cosmetic surgeon, I can tell you that photographs, even in a perfect state, tell very little about your level of vitality and attractiveness—because so much of that, both objective and subjective, comes through the dynamic kinetic emotions and the way you carry yourself in live action.

Pro-aging means you should relish the communities that social media and the internet can create for you, but also be discerning in your use of social media when it comes to your goals and needs. Stop comparing yourself to the filtered, altered, and fake photos you see on Instagram. Those friends and celebrities you're following don't look that good in real life. Trust me. I know—they're my patients!

Put Your Electronic Devices Away—You Already Know This, Don't You?

How do we stop obsessing about our cringe-worthy selfies?

By putting the electronics away.

I'm sure you know by now that if you want to have a restful night's sleep, you need to shut off all the electronics—phones, computers, tablets—for at least an hour before bedtime. Electronic screens emit blue light, which is approximately one-third of all the visible light emitted by the sun. As in, the wavelength of light that wakes you up! This means your brain is being stimulated, even if you're watching something relaxing.

We are addicted to our devices, and I'm as guilty as most people. On weekends, my fingers start to twitch if I'm not picking up my phone and returning an email, but I know that if I don't put the devices away, I'm going to regret the time I didn't spend with my family as soon as I get back to the office on Monday. So I force myself to be disciplined about my electronics when I'm not at the office unless, of course, it's a medical emergency. I know that, 99 percent of the time, the messages I'm getting on my phone do *not* need to be addressed until the morning.

Don't be afraid of being less productive because you've shut down your email for a few hours. Spend time interacting with what is live and in front of you, even if it's just the view. You have to believe that scheduling that time off will make you better than anybody else. Look at these people you think are so successful—they're scattered and frazzled and unproductive precisely because they never shut down!"

Putting the electronics away is not only a good way to connect with the real people in your community, but to reconnect with yourself. Because one of the best things you can do for yourself is to do what I grew up doing: nothing! Or rather, give yourself the opportunity to tune out the chatter, and daydream. Which is the root of all creativity.

I know this because, if you're concentrating on a message or something else, you're not in your head. When cellphones became popular and email a way of life, we all told ourselves they would make our lives more efficient and productive, and we'd have more downtime to spend with our loved ones or doing the things we like. But what do we do instead? Spend so much time on our devices that we have no time left for anything else.

This reminds me of something the contemporary spiritual teacher and author Eckhart Tolle said. If someone kept him waiting and apologized for it, Tolle said to them there was nothing to be sorry for, because he wasn't waiting; he was just *being*. That's really it. Allow yourself to just *be*. So much more work can be accomplished by doing that than by returning a few emails or checking Twitter. Let your brain get the reset it needs!

This also reminds me of when I was a child, and I remember being bored a lot. It's not that my parents didn't offer me plenty of options to keep me busy, but I wasn't athletic, so I wasn't caught up in sports or teams or summer camp or many of the things that my peers were doing. I still have vivid and pleasurable memories of riding the school bus and leaning my head against the window and watching the world go by. Daydreaming about nothing in particular and sometimes even dozing off. Funnily enough now, when people tell me they're bored, I laugh and tell them that I'd pay for some boredom now, so I could have the time to just sit with myself.

You know I'm right. Put those devices away and reconnect with the real world!

Community Is What Keeps You Young

Play Young and Feel Young

I am in awe of my son who, as a young teenager, is a whiz at swimming and surfing and running track, especially as I was so totally uninterested in anything athletic until I discovered roller skating. He is learning, early on, as I eventually did, that athletic and/or creative endeavors during those crucial developmental years are transformative. They give children and teens positive reinforcement, self-awareness, valuable physical skills, and, most important, a sense of accomplishment and camaraderie from teamwork. From being part of that community.

The point here is that being young and feeling young requires that you stay and continually engage in the journey through the actions of learning, filtering, aspiring, and growing. This journey doesn't end. You don't just grow up and then grow old. The concept of community, and the one you are constantly building for yourself, is one of the most essential components of pro-aging.

Spend Time with People Who Care

Whether you're online in the virtual world or engaging in the real world, it is essential to pay attention to things that can give back to you. Staring at the images of Photoshopped celebrities or the super wealthy on their private jets posted on social media is not serving you or your self-image or anyone. The emotional scale is not balanced. Looking at your out-of-town best friend's new baby photos may serve you better. Planning a trip to see her will do the same.

All relationships must serve a role; there must be give and take. Although all relationships wax and wane, the overall trajectory must be in your best interest. Even in our most altruistic moments, these activities make us feel good about ourselves. Resist the activities, the people, the news, the commercialism, and the thought patterns that don't serve you. Awareness of what serves you best is the most important step—and the ideal way to find it is with people who care.

> *Awareness of what serves you best is the most important step—and the ideal way to find it is with people who care.*

Resist the Negative, Manifest the Positive

It's really about whom you surround yourself with. We all collect baggage and accumulate garbage as we get older—people and influences and things—and they're not always the best. We attach to routines. It can get to a point where we get into an unhealthy cycle of feast and famine, not just with food, but with every aspect of our lives. When that happens, a clutter clean-out is desperately needed. Otherwise, you won't be pro-aging. You'll just be aging.

Which is why one thing I have learned as a physician and as a husband, father, and member of my community is that, as we get older, we need to surround ourselves with things that are positive, rather than negative. Embrace your community. Embrace your friends and loved ones. Make a phone call to someone you care about every day before you start your workday. (I speak to my dad almost every morning on the way to work.) Spend a few minutes highlighting and thinking about the things you have and like, both physically and materially. Avoid negative bashing of people or ideas or gossip; rather, engage in the promotion of things you do believe in and be resolution-focused of people or situations that are distasteful. If that is not possible, avoid those things or those people.

No matter how connected you are, no matter how in touch with yourself, no matter how much you strive to do the right thing, it's also okay when you're off-balance. It happens. Everyone has days when they go off-kilter. Instead of beating yourself up about it—which just compounds the worry and releases more of the stress hormones that make you look drawn and subpar—accept it. It's all part of the process. The off-days teach you about how to get to and how to appreciate the balanced days. Things can always change for better or worse in a split second. There is no doubt that staying positive will always help tip those scales.

PART TWO

NOURISH YOUR INSIDE

CHAPTER 6

Eliminating the Extrinsic Evildoers of Aging

You can't help getting older,
but you don't have to get old.

—GEORGE BURNS

Genetic destiny is something no one can control. But some of the most potent factors that contribute to aging—you know what I mean: smoking, drinking/drugs, sugar/junk food, and too much sun—are more firmly in your grasp.

We live in a world that is more stressful and complicated than previous generations. That's why we're sold detoxification and why wellness is such a huge marketing issue. In my opinion, however, the wellness community is not a reflection of healthier living. It's exactly the opposite, a reflection instead that we're living our lives on the brink and burning our candles at both ends. We invented cellphones and computers to save us time, but they've actually given us less time and more work to do, with higher expectations.

So I totally understand why these evildoers of aging are an essential part of people's lives. For me, life without an occasional martini when I want one, or a chocolate-chip cookie when I'm craving one, would be no fun at all! One of my weaknesses is that I tend to be a feast-or-famine person. When I go on vacation, I eat everything and drink a little alcohol every day. Then I come back home, and I go back to a strict pro-aging routine. Some people are better at moderation than others.

We build a tolerance to everything that ages us, and the more we do it, the more we want it. The sooner you start pro-aging, cutting back in small steps, the better your results will be. You can protect yourself against the toxicity you may not even realize is in your world once you know what to look for.

1. Toxicity

"Toxins" is one of those buzzwords that is overused and over-hyped, because most people don't understand what is actually "toxic" or not.

Toxins are things that interfere with the healthful biological functions of your body. They set you back by either killing living cells or altering cellular activity in a detrimental way. Pollution, certain chemicals and pesticides, and even medicines are examples.

How to Undo Toxicity: The Truth Behind Detoxing

The concept of detoxification, or "freeing yourself of toxins," is sold to us in the wellness media, as is the belief that every disease and anything bad that happens to us is a result of a toxin. Every cancer, every bad mood, every bowel movement is a result of some toxin that must be extracted with the aid of supplements or colonics or other treatments. That, I'm here to tell you, is a crock.

It is nothing more than modern-era exorcisms similar to the days when religion preceded science and demons were the cause of all wrongdoings and illness.

You don't need a juicer or a "cleanse" or expensive supplements to "get the toxins out." Your body already has an amazing built-in detox system, thanks to the ceaseless filters provided by your detox organs—your liver and kidneys. These sophisticated self-defense mechanisms deal with toxins and keep you alive. Your liver and kidneys filter what you take in and ingest every day. They clearly don't work all the time, as toxins can build up and cause us humans enormous detriment, but they are not the cause of every disease, and they are most certainly not all fixable by the varying techniques sold to us every day.

There is *nothing* we can put into our body to extract toxins themselves, unless you have a disease state and/or have been poisoned by substances such as mercury, lead, or other metals. (This is called chelation therapy.)

The best way to detoxify your body is not to ingest any toxins in the first place.

So you can stop thinking about toxins like the demon in *The Exorcist*! The best way to detoxify your body is not to ingest any toxins in the first place.When people claim that they feel better after a "juice cleanse," it's not the juicing that's doing it. It's the stepping away from what you normally would have eaten during the "cleanse." And even though we live in a world saturated with artificial substances, we can optimize our body's filtration system by being cautious about what we eat and drink. This means cutting back on fake and processed foods, on excessive amounts of any one type of real food, and on pharmaceuticals, in general. It means ensuring that our homes circulate fresh air. It means not using pesticides or herbicides on our lawns and gardens or fruits and vegetables. It means knowing where our meats and dairy come from.

Detoxifying skin treatments sold to consumers can be equally confusing. There are enormous paradoxes in the skincare industry, such as oxygen infusion facials versus antioxidant therapies. Is oxygen a bad or a good thing? The answer is complex but like most things, it's neither good nor bad; it's all about balance. What is consistent is that something always gets a positive spin when it's being sold to us, or a negative spin when someone is selling its antidote.

Remember: the body is an imperfect machine and we, as humans, were never meant to live as long as we now do. Despite your liver and kidneys doing their best, there's going to be a higher rate of everything as we age, including chronic disease.

But even when your body is imperfect, it's still an amazing machine. Everything we do in architecture and engineering is trying to mimic what the universe has already created in the human form. The greatest engine that humans could make would have something like 30 percent fuel efficiency—nowhere close to that of the mitochondria in a human cell.

Be a smart consumer and stop wasting your time on "cleanses" and "detoxes." Everything that's potentially good can also be potentially bad. You have to learn to avoid the hype and step back. Allow your body to reset. It's amazing how your body can do that. Eat a good diet and move your body and allow it to do the job that a million years of evolution have taught it to do. Those are the best detoxes in the world.

2. Smoking

We all know that smoking is worse than bad. If you're about to have surgery, it dramatically affects healing, causing more bleeding and scarring. It's carcinogenic and addictive and wholly toxic.

According to the Centers for Disease Control, smoking kills over 7 million people around the world each year and "is responsible for more than 480,000 deaths per year in the United States, including more than 41,000 deaths resulting from secondhand smoke exposure. This is about one in five deaths annually, or 1,300 deaths every day. On average, smokers die ten years earlier than nonsmokers."

There have been numerous studies showing the effects of smoking on identical twins, where only one was a smoker. By the time the twins hit fifty, they look like completely different people. I can tell a patient who's a heavy smoker by the fact that they tend to look older than their years, since smoking speeds up the aging process. From dullness of skin tone to fine lines and wrinkles to sagginess, smoking breaks down every layer and every luminous quality you want your skin to have.

Smoking affects the health of blood vessels and the therefore the blood supply throughout the entire body, including the skin. Collagen is found in every single blood vessel, and smoking breaks it down.

Don't be fooled by marketing for ultra-light, additive-free, or organic cigarettes. They're still made from tobacco and they're still equally toxic. And, while vaping doesn't contain the multitude of toxins that tobacco does, it still contains nicotine, as well as potentially toxic chemicals to transport the nicotine, and flavors. It's not yet fully known how it affects the lungs, circulatory system, or skin when inhaled. We're just starting to see the health consequences for the vaping generation.

How to Undo Smoking

The biggest problem for smokers, as you likely know, is that nicotine is an extremely addictive drug, and the addiction is extremely difficult to break.

For those who are serious about quitting, sometimes having a health scare or fears of lung cancer will do the trick. Others are worried about their increased risk of heart attack and stroke. Anecdotally, I've found that people who see graphic photos of what smoking does to *skin* are more likely to quit than those who see photos of diseased lungs.

Thanks to your body's amazing resilience, and, as discussed above, its reparative capacity, many studies have shown that if you stop smoking for ten to fifteen years—no matter how much you smoked before then, or for how long—your risk of lung and other cancers goes down dramatically, nearly to levels of someone who's never smoked. Fortunately, the smoking rates have gone down in the US, mostly due to public-space laws limiting the potential to smoke. Clearly, the less people see others smoking, the less likely they are to do it; like any habit, negative or positive, there is certainly social reinforcement for it. Surrounding yourself with nonsmokers is certainly a good and effective incentive to quit. This holds true of any behavior. I always recommend that people surround themselves with those who have the attributes they aspire toward, whether healthy eaters, nonsmokers, or athletic people. Positivity, like negativity, is contagious. This is why our parents wanted us hanging out with the "good kids," and why we should always be cautious of whom we surround ourselves.

3. Drinking

Many of my male patients come to me for help getting rid of their puffy eyes and blotchy and dull complexion. They sometimes admit that drinking wine or having a couple of cocktails every night is their only vice, and they're crestfallen when I have to tell them that these very same drinks are what brought them into my office. Because when you take away the "in" and "ation" from intoxication, all you're left with is *toxic*.

By definition, that's what drinking alcohol is: you are intoxicating your body. That feeling of relaxation or being buzzed or drunk or wasted or anything along the spectrum of being mentally and physically altered by the drug alcohol is a form of neurologic intoxication. You're not getting a release of the feel-good neurochemicals like the serotonin and dopamine that you get when you exercise or when you're in love. You're getting toxified, and as that happens, the alcohol is altering and often damaging your brain cells and your liver cells, and over the long term, it's causing a whole lot of other problems.

> *Despite a false common perception that alcohol is good for you, the safest amount of alcohol you can drink is precisely zero.*

Despite a false common perception that alcohol is good for you, the safest amount of alcohol you can drink is precisely zero. Sorry, kids, your heart isn't healthier because of red wine. This false belief shouldn't be reinforcing daily alcohol consumption. If you want to drink, drink. I do. But knowing what it does to me helps me regulate my drinking. It also helps me enlighten patients when they reach a level of frustration, one that is often caused not just by their affinity for alcohol, but merely by the amounts they often falsely see as benign.

People drink to reach whatever level of intoxication they seek. Yes, it's a form of relaxation that might be mild and relaxing from one flavorful glass of red wine, but that lovely buzz is still caused by neurochemical effects on your brain. In fact, alcohol does a number on nearly every organ in the body. One of its main metabolites after being broken down by the enzyme alcohol dehydrogenase is acetaldehyde, a potent and toxic chemical. You've heard of the hangover, right? You can thank this chemical for that.

Like smoking, drinking also adversely affects the heart and liver, and is a huge risk factor for developing several cancers.

Alcohol often causes shifts in metabolism, leading to weight gain. It also weakens your immune system and limits the functions of your detoxifying organs, the liver and kidneys, causing a double whammy of toxic effects. Like smoking, alcohol use and abuse are some of the largest contributors to preventable disease in our nation, and to with the financial burden on our healthcare system. As for your skin, alcohol clearly causes premature aging.

In past generations, there have been studies about the "health benefits of red wine" or "moderate drinking," but this research tends to be funded by alcohol companies and spread by their lobbyists. These lobbyists also capitalize on the common misperceptions about what moderate or heavy drinking is. These figures will always be faulty and overgeneralized, because how well your body metabolizes alcohol is based on your height and weight along with other genetic factors. (If you're 5' 10", you could process more than somebody who's 5' 0".)

According to the US Department of Health and Human Services, moderate drinking is up to one drink per day for women and up to two drinks per day for men. (Can men really drink twice as much and not have negative effects as compared to women? I somehow doubt that.) A shot of vodka or other spirits, a six-ounce glass of wine, or a twelve-ounce can of beer is considered one drink. Women who have more than seven drinks a week are considered *heavy* drinkers! My patients are shocked when I tell them that. I can see them calculating how many drinks they had when they went out to dinner—a few glasses of champagne, perhaps, and a few glasses of wine, and then a couple of cocktails with friends or their partners every week. Maybe they will have four drinks on two nights, and several drinks the other nights of the week. They feel that if they don't get drunk, then, surely, they can't be heavy drinkers.

As with food, there are individual metabolic differences and ethnic variations that affect how well you process alcohol. As you get older, your metabolic activity goes down, which makes it harder on your liver. Toxic effects obviously increase with age, in case you're wondering why you don't recover like you used to. Over time, the toxic effects of alcohol are similar, whether you're a heavy drinker or a moderate drinker. It's a matter of severity. Clearly, no one categorizes or talks about light drinkers who have one to three drinks per week. No one does because they are not worth marketing to. To the alcohol industry, they are passive drinkers, practically nondrinkers. So why do any research on them?

Your liver is very smart and always working. After a night of several drinks, your liver enzymes rise significantly as a result of its efforts to deal with the alcohol. The more you toxify it, the more it works, and it builds its resistance. People who drink every day tend not to get drunk on two glasses of wine at dinner. Their liver accommodates after being stressed. But—and this is a *big* but!—people think that because they've developed a high tolerance for drinking, it means that they're not getting the negative effect of alcohol. They think that, because they're not intoxicated, there's no toxic effect on their bodies. Sadly, they're wrong. The negative effects of alcohol are cumulative.

I've known many moderate to heavy drinkers that practice a month a year of zero alcohol consumption. As soon as these people start drinking again, though, they get intoxicated quickly. In only a month, their livers had detoxified and lost their compensatory tolerance. It's amazing how quickly our bodies can adjust.

My theory is: no alcohol is best, but we do have to live our lives—we supposedly only go around once, right? I certainly indulged throughout my younger years, when I had greater resilience and recovery. We have to find the balance for ourselves. I merely want to impart knowledge to help you do that, so being straightforward about the most widely accepted form of toxification in the world is, I believe, a worthy conversation to have. I don't mean to be a spoilsport—you will rarely see me turn down a drink at a social event if I don't have to work the next day. But as I have gotten older, my ability to process alcohol has, like most people's, dramatically changed. I still enjoy alcohol, but, clearly, the balance has shifted as my tolerance of its negative consequences has diminished greatly. And, in most circumstances, I prefer to feel good when I wake in the morning. Alcohol impedes this, along with the ability to maximize all other aspects of my life, such as my exercise tolerance, my diet, my quality of work, my sleep, and, most important, my self-perception, either in the mirror or between my ears. This is why, over the years, I have gone from being a moderate drinker to a very light one.

How to Decrease Drinking

Studies show that, if you stop entirely or dramatically decrease drinking, your liver, other organs, and especially your skin repair themselves. I have never encountered a single patient who took a long hiatus from drinking who didn't tell me it has improved the way they look, how they feel, and how they function.

If this is where you say, "But I love to drink. I don't want to give that up," I would say it's your prerogative not to change a thing habitually. Do what makes you happy, as long as you do no harm to anyone. But consider this distinct possibility: if you're willing to concede that you may just be happier if you dramatically reduce your alcohol intake for the mere reason that it is clearly a toxifying depressant that is simply not that good for you or your potential to feel and look your best...then it might be time to cut back or stop drinking altogether.

What works for me, as I've explained, is to very rarely drink during the work week, and then have a few drinks on weekends, if I feel like it. As a result, my tolerance is very low, so this is enough for me to enjoy the relaxing effect of the alcohol and feel as if I'm partying like it's 1999. If I drink more than that, I feel it. It's not that I feel awful or even hungover, but I'm not the best version of myself. If that's something you're considering, pick two days (just two) to have a couple of drinks. On those days, enjoy the alcohol but don't binge; for the rest of the week, stick to water! I drink sparkling water with a splash of cranberry juice and a lime at weekday events, or I order a glass of wine and maybe take a sip or two and let it sit. I generally don't want those around me to feel uncomfortable if I don't drink—which, oddly, people do. And if there's a week when I don't drink at all, I don't double up the next week as I know my mind, liver, and skin will pay the price.

Let me leave you with this sobering fact: Alcohol is one of the largest causes of morbidity and mortality in this country. It's a huge burden for the economy, the healthcare industry, and family members who have to deal with the fallout of alcohol abuse. Enjoy it when you consume it in small amounts—but realize that the more you drink, the more you need to drink to get that feeling of enjoyment. If you want to be the best version of yourself, respect the toxicity of alcohol for what it is. Take it seriously. You'll be a lot better at pro-aging when you do.

A Few Words About Drugs

Not all mind-altering drugs are toxic, and not all toxic drugs are illegal. But many readily available drugs, legal and illegal, can have a toxic effect on your behavior that puts you in harm's way and, at the very least, minimize your potential. Any regular impairment of judgment can lead people astray.

We live in a world of pharmaceutical intervention and self-medication. Clearly, with such catastrophes as the opioid crisis, the system is rigged to maximize profits and satisfy a population looking for quick fixes like antidepressants, anti-anxiety meds, painkillers, and prescription amphetamines. It is not within the scope of this book to recommend for or against the use of any prescription medications. They all clearly exist for legitimate reasons. Sadly, a significant portion of society is addicted to one type of drug or another, legal or illegal, and with or without a valid diagnosis. It is only my general recommendation to minimize pharmaceuticals as a whole, particularly ones that alter judgment or perception. For every action, there is a reaction.

When intervention is needed, whether it be for high blood pressure, high cholesterol, depression, or any cosmetic malady, I always suggest maximizing the beneficial means of healthy living and self-motivation first. The primary and most important steps with any health issue start from within. Only then can we truly benefit from whatever treatments or pharmaceuticals modern medicine has to offer.

4. Sugar and Junk Food

I have to confess that one of my weaknesses is for chocolate chip cookies. Insomnia Cookies is a bakery in New York City that was created just for people like me—you call them, and twenty minutes later, there are cookies delivered to your door. Fortunately for my blood sugar, they don't deliver to my address, but when the cravings hit, I have been known to get in an Uber with my son to make a cookie run. Do I feel bad about this? No, yes, maybe, sometimes. Does it stop me from going? What do you think?

Frankly, I think that sugar should be classified as an addictive drug, because our taste buds have been primed to crave it—it is why the food industry does everything in its power to keep on tempting those taste buds so you keep buying stuff you know you shouldn't. The junk food bombarding us in every aisle of the grocery store is so laden with sugar that it's hard to know when something tastes really sweet anymore. It's everywhere it's not really needed—like in our cereal, peanut better, protein bars, yogurt, ketchup, granola bars, and "power" drinks.

In his book *10 Minutes/10 Years*, published in 2007, cosmetic dermatologist Dr. Fredric Brandt, one of my many mentors, was one of the first dermatologists to write about how sugar causes inflammation, which has a negative effect not only on your health, but on your skin. He discussed endogenous glycation, "a natural process where sugar molecules in the blood and in the cells chemically bond to protein fibers and DNA, changing their shape and properties...in the process eventually forming harmful new molecules called advanced glycation products." These molecules are what's responsible for the inflammatory effect, especially on collagen, which is the most prevalent protein in your body. They cause the collagen to become brittle—and lead to wrinkles, sagging, and a loss of resilience.

Sugar doesn't just come in the form of white table sugar, candy, or processed foods. Your body converts all refined carbohydrates like white bread, white rice, white pasta, and fruit juice, to glucose (or blood sugar), causing insulin spikes that lead to an almost immediate release of these inflammatory compounds. Clearly, sugar is one of the pro-aging enemies.

How to Undo Sugar/Junk Food Consumption

Start reading labels, so you can stop purchasing any foods that contain hidden sugars. Learn to recognize some of the trick names (like maltodextrin, date sugar, fructose, or turbinado) that might make you think the sugar in that food is somehow healthier. There's no such thing as a good or bad sugar—raw organic cane sugar certainly sounds healthier than high-fructose corn syrup, but the corn syrup is super concentrated, so you need more of the cane sugar to get the same taste. But they're both still just sugar.

Reducing sugar-laden foods can help. I know this is hard for people to believe, but when you start cutting back on sugar, you honestly lose your taste for it, so when you do eat something sweet, it's almost like it sets your teeth on edge!

I eat fruit when I want something sweet. I consider refined carbohydrates like pasta or bread to be a dessert, even though they aren't "sweet"—meaning that they're more of a treat instead of part of my regular, healthy, pro-aging meal. If I'm eating out and the server brings a basket of some wonderful fresh-baked bread, I'll eat the bread and not have dessert. If I skip the bread, I might split a dessert with my fellow guests.

I also make a conscious effort to eat only fresh desserts. I believe that homemade ice cream, homemade whipped cream, and homemade chocolate cake have got to be better than a packaged cake mix or a cheap bar of chocolate.

5. Sun Exposure

Do you know the story of margarine? It was invented in 1869 by a French chemist for those who couldn't afford butter, and over the years it evolved from the French version (made with beef fat and water) to the American version of vegetable oils processed into a bar or a tub. When I was growing up, I was taught that margarine made from vegetable oil was healthier than butter. Years later, we now know that the hardening process, using high temperatures to heat liquid vegetable oils, can be extremely unhealthy for your heart and metabolism.

So what does margarine have to do with the sun? Well, it has to do with scientists and society telling us one thing...and then finding out, years later, that that one thing was wrong. Harmful, even. These historical contradictions are very common in science and society. Nothing is 100 percent set in stone, so stay open-minded. As one of my mentors, Dr. Rhoda Narins, used to tell me: "Believe half of what you see and none of what you read."

Controversy exists among scientists and dermatologists in the current discussion around sun exposure. Beyond using sunscreen, I want to talk about how much sun exposure is needed for a healthy pro-aging body. Let me preface this section by saying that, first and foremost, I'm a dermatologist, and sun exposure is a known problem. It causes skin cancer and it *will* damage your skin over time. I am, by no means, giving you permission to go bake in the sun unprotected.

That said, I am not in the camp of demonizing all sun exposure, like many of my dermatological colleagues. Ironically, even dermatologists who are very anti-sun still prescribe artificial ultraviolet light exposure for chronic skin diseases, such as eczema and psoriasis. Sunlight clearly has an anti-inflammatory and immune-modulatory impact. We also know there is a very real problem for those who get little sunlight in winter months—called SAD (seasonal affective disorder), a type of depression with a recurring seasonal pattern. Along with medication and psychotherapy, the most common treatment for SAD is light therapy. Clearly, sunlight affects mood.

Obviously, if the sun has some sort of therapeutic benefit for people with skin diseases and/or SAD, why shouldn't it have some holistic benefit, at the right dose, for everyone else? There have been studies showing that people who live outdoor lives and are exposed to more sunlight have less heart disease and better blood pressure, thought to be a result of the sun-stimulated production of nitric oxide, a potent vasodilator. Naysayers would claim this would be due to their getting more exercise than sedentary office workers.

The key to this argument is trying to understand what is a "healthy" versus an "unhealthy" dose of sunlight to make you feel good, be healthy, and not trigger potential cancers or skin damage. We'll never be able to figure that out if we're so closed-minded that we tell all people of all races and colors to live in the shade and only venture into bright sunlight when clad in protective clothing, gobs of sunscreen, and a wide-brimmed hat, particularly in the US.

> *One in five people in the world will have a nonmelanoma skin cancer in their lifetime.*

Still, skin cancer is directly correlated to sun exposure. One thing we know for sure is that UVA and UVB rays are carcinogenic. One in five people in the world will have a nonmelanoma skin cancer in their lifetime. Melanoma is increasing around the world, especially in younger populations, and it's a bit more controversial than other skin cancers, as there is a huge genetic component, and many people often get it in non-sun-exposed areas.

With skin cancer rates on the rise, some dermatologists and researchers have a theory that, ironically, *sunscreen* may be one of the reasons behind the increase—because most people don't use it properly, have a false sense of security about sun exposure, and end up getting far less protection than they think. It is true that most people don't know how to apply sunscreen. They don't put it on at least twenty to thirty minutes before going outside, so they're basically unprotected until it becomes activated. They apply it unevenly, and they forget to reapply it.

Other studies have shown that people who have chronic, regular exposure to the sun (like sailors or farmers)—a condition called hardening—may be less likely to develop melanoma than those who have intermittent sun exposure and a tendency to burn. There *may* be a protective therapeutic element to mild and constant sun exposure due to protective melanin, but this hypothesis is certainly not license to go bake on the beach.

I've always felt that you can't just categorize sunlight as bad for everybody, and the current sun-exposure guidelines don't take into account the variety of skin tones that exist. Dermatology can actually be a racist field; we must pass medical judgment based on skin color, so we can't tell people who are African-American and less prone to sunburns—and very rarely get melanoma—to treat their skin the same as Caucasian people who get freckles and burn every time they go to the beach.

All life on earth comes from the sun. Humans evolved as outdoor creatures, and our bodies still need *some* amount of sun exposure—even if it's a mere few minutes a day. The sun has an amazing immune-regulatory effect, as well as positive effects on our well-being, especially in the synthesis of vitamin D. Without vitamin D, we are at a clear risk for a weakened immune system and a host of diseases. While real food sources make up the majority of needed vitamin D, studies are revealing that, even though supplements make your bloodwork numbers go up, they don't change the actual biologic detriments of vitamin D deficiency. Some amount of sunlight is essential.

Once again, history is changing its opinion on supplements of all kinds. That doesn't mean you should get excited about baring your skin at the beach all day. It really doesn't take that much sunlight to get your daily dose of vitamin D—maybe ten or fifteen minutes' worth, on about 15 percent of your body. The point is that nothing is generally all bad or all good. Time, social trends, and science change our viewpoint on everything over the years. My theory is to educate then customize, both for myself and my patients. Cautious moderation is always a good technique for anything pro-aging.

How to Undo Excessive Sun Exposure

Hiding in the shade and wearing sun-protective clothing all the time is an unrealistic goal for most of the population. We are meant to be outdoors. I love the beach and outdoor sports, and I wear sunscreen. I love the feeling of sunlight on my face.

But do I lie in the sun to get tan? I do *not*. I find it a huge pain to coat myself every hour or two with SPF 30 sunscreen, so I take walks and play sports on the beach, either early in the morning or after 3:30 p.m. I have a long lunch and read in the shade during the sun's peak danger hours. I can enjoy the feeling of heat on my skin, and I only have to put on sunscreen a few times throughout the day. I don't have to worry about being outside because I know that I'm not overdoing it.

In my opinion, moving your body and being outdoors are very important for optimal health, particularly for people like me who work in an office all day. If you get a mild to moderate amount of sunlight, depending on the amount of exposed skin that you've protected with sunscreen, I don't think you have to worry that it's going to be life-threatening. Authorities in Australia and New Zealand, two countries where skin cancer rates are among the highest in the world, agree with this stance, and their guidelines about sun exposure have recently changed because scientists there believe that *some* sunlight exposure is therapeutic. Unless the UV index is above three, Australia doesn't even recommend daily sunscreen. Scientists also recommend a few minutes a day of exposure for health benefits. The US is not this open-minded.

That doesn't mean you should bake on the beach all day with no sunscreen on. If you're at any high risk, such as having very fair skin, a family history of skin cancer, a prior history of skin cancer, or if you're worried about anything whatsoever, see a dermatologist. You should probably see one every year anyway for a comprehensive skin check.

Use sunscreen. Stay out of direct sunlight during the peak hours. Live your life. When I spend the day at the beach or come back from vacation, I always feel healthier. It's not just being relaxed, and it's not the heat or the fresh salt air if I've been at the beach. It's the *sunlight*.

CHAPTER 7

The Pro-Aging Way to Eat

One cannot think well, love well, sleep well,
if one has not dined well.

—VIRGINIA WOOLF

A healthy weight is very important for pro-agers—and for everyone, of course.

That can be hard to maintain because we've turned sustenance into a drug. When it comes to food, we often confuse what we *need* with what we *want*. In addition, it's often hard to know the difference between *how* we eat and what we think we need—so much food is put in front of us when we go out to eat or order takeout that it's really hard to know what a serving size is anymore.

This isn't made any easier by food fads and diets du jour, and our own health authorities changing their minds about what's healthy or not. Remember when low-fat was all the rage, and suddenly there were fat-free items everywhere? But what was the fat replaced with? Sugar. That just made us hungrier and fatter.

Being at a healthy weight depends on many factors. Our bodies have an approximate preset figure that might be under or over what society considers ideal, which puts enormous pressure on too many people to yo-yo up and down the scale.

I still remember being teased as a "husky" child. Those days are long gone, and I now closely watch what I eat. I generally don't buy junk food, and I always have unsweetened foods, raw veggies and hummus, and an assortment of nuts and whole grains in the office and at home. My dietary habits are best described as Mediterranean: lots of fruit, vegetables, nuts, and fish. I consider refined carbohydrates and all sugars as treats, and I have come to believe that maintaining my weight isn't just about good eating habits, but about good eating *timing*.

An important way to pro-age is by rethinking food. Here is my disclosure: I am not a registered dietician; I have not written books on the subject prior to this; nor am I a supermodel influencer selling a holistic nutritional lifestyle. I am physician—one who throughout his life has had issues with food. As a medical leader in the various surgical and nonsurgical techniques of fat removal, I have had the opportunity, during twenty years of experience, to hear about my patients' struggles with dietary habits, to educate myself, and to consult with some of the smartest people in the nutrition industry.

In this chapter, you will hear from leading experts in the field of nutrition, along with some of my own anecdotal experiences and research into the various perspectives and means of controlling our weight and using food to make us look good, to feel good, and to live a pro-aging lifestyle.

It's Not *What* You Eat, But *When* You Eat

Once you change the *timing* of when you eat, you may realize that you're less hungry *and* you're no longer mindlessly snacking, so you'll eat less and maintain weight more easily without even thinking about it.

The Power of Fast Mimicking

Every major religion incorporates some form of fasting into its practices—for spiritual reasons and for purification. There are basic fasts, where you eat nothing for a certain period; restrictive fasts (such as juice fasts), where you eat or drink only one type of food; intermittent fasts, where you eat within a limited time period each day; and fast mimicking, where you eat a very low amount of calories for a few days only.

I was introduced to the concept of fasting for health when I read about the work of Dr. Valter Longo, PhD, director of the program on longevity and cancer at the IFOM research center in Milan, Italy, and director of the Institute of Longevity at the Davis School of Gerontology at the University of Southern California in Los Angeles. His theory and research maintain that restricting your caloric intake for a short period of time, no more than five days—what's called fast mimicking—puts our bodies in *repair mode*. It cleanses and improves our physical and mental well-being by allowing our bodies to do their work properly; it resets both the metabolic and psychological reliance we have on the things we tend to overdo nutritionally. His research also suggests the role of fast mimicking in improving chronic conditions that involve inflammation, which is just about all diseases. Whether a one-time jumpstart or a practice done several times a year, I have found fast mimicking to be groundbreaking in its pro-aging role.

Funnily enough, fast mimicking is one of the few things in my theory of pro-aging that goes against my belief that there's no such thing as "dieting"—because we all know that diets usually don't work. Pro-aging is about making small adjustments, restructuring habits as we age, and slow and steady increments that add up over the long term. But this very short-term, periodic fasting jolt makes a big difference in how well your body functions. It also gives you the psychological jolt you might need to make further changes in your attitude toward what, how, when, and why you eat.

I do fast mimicking by buying Dr. Longo's ready-made, limited-calorie meal kit, called ProLon (I receive zero sponsorship for using this product). The first day is 1,000 calories as you get eased in; by the second day, you're down to 600; and by the fifth day, you're at 500 calories. I've found that, although there are periods of hunger, I always find the second day the hardest. But you're never starving. You eat something every few hours. A high fluid intake is deliberate, and I've found that I drink a lot more than usual, as I get very thirsty. This helps curb your appetite as well. I've also noticed that, during the five days, you need to go to the bathroom with increased frequency.

I schedule my fast mimicking three times a year; the recommendation is two or three times each year for the typical healthy adult, and more often for particularly inflammatory or other health conditions. (If you can't afford the meal kit, or want to create your own plan, you can research the topic and improvise.) I choose to do fast mimicking after the winter holidays, a vacation, or a personal celebration where I ate and drank more than usual (enjoying every moment of it, of course!), and feel the need to get back on track. Going through a period of fasting has the potential to give enormous psychological clarity and physical endurance. It always works at resetting and recharging my body, so I go back to my normal eating pattern without feeling the need to binge.

I must add that fast mimicking works extremely well for me, but it may not work well for others; no technique works for everyone. But the clinical research is there, and it is a growing trend based on historical traditions and modern science. Many of my patients with whom I have shared the experience and research have found success with it as well.

In addition, some people should *never* do fast mimicking, including those with certain illnesses or medical conditions such as diabetes, and those who don't have a high enough percentage of fat in their bodies. Consulting with a nutritionist or healthcare professionals specializing in metabolic diseases may be necessary before you start any fast-mimicking program.

Intermittent Fasting: The Eight-Hour Eating Schedule

While fast mimicking isn't meant to be done very often, intermittent fasting is generally how I eat every day, with some leeway. When done strictly, it has proven to be an excellent weight-loss and/or maintenance technique for many people. I hope it will become as powerful a pro-aging strategy for you as it has become for me.

Intermittent fasting means that you eat all your meals, including snacks, within an eight-hour period. It isn't about restricting calories, although, of course, it's not a license to gorge. Instead, it's about optimizing and regulating your metabolism—because calories are *not* all the same.

You might be wondering if this contradicts the science that says to eat something healthy every two hours to keep your metabolism up. Yes, it does, but that's because your metabolism is circadian; it acts differently at different times of the day. Obviously, eating within an hour of bedtime (or in the middle of the night) is different than having an early dinner, right? The body likes a regular rhythm; it likes consistency; and it functions best on routine. That doesn't mean we can't challenge ourselves with food like we do with exercise. But in regard to nutrition, timing is of the essence. This is because there are different metabolic effects, depending on what time you're eating the same food. In other words, a sandwich at lunchtime is not processed by your body the same way as the very same sandwich you might eat right before bed. *When* you eat your food has a huge impact on what your body does with those calories.

If you do a lot of research, you will find, as I did, that we've been sold the notion that breakfast is the most important meal of the day. Who sells that? Breakfast-food companies.

Everyone's circadian rhythms are different, including mine. I am almost never hungry enough to eat a meal when I get up, and I usually don't eat more than one hundred calories before noon, most days. I like to get up and go. In fact, I wouldn't eat at all in the morning if I didn't exercise, but I need a little bit of energy in my body to get me through my pre-office workout.

Another reason intermittent fasting is powerful is that it clues you in to your stress-eating patterns. It isn't just about switching your meal timing, it's about learning to recognize hunger and triggers for snacks or comfort foods. When you know you can only eat within a prescribed period, your body eventually stops wanting snacks, like the mindless ones at night. If you don't believe me, try it! It takes a bit of concentrated effort to set up a different eating schedule, but once you get used to it, it's surprisingly easy. If I first eat a real meal at noon, then I will finish eating by 8:00 p.m.

What do you do when you have a demanding work schedule and find it hard to stick to the eight-hour rule? There are exceptions to every rule, of course. I have friends who, when they know they're going out to dinner later, will eat around 1:00 p.m. so they can be finished with dinner by 9:00 p.m. Whereas they'd normally eat around 10:00 a.m. and have dinner at 6:00 p.m. And, as you know, if you're going out for a meal, whether for work or for pleasure, and it's off your schedule, enjoy it. You know my philosophy by now: Don't cheat—treat!

Supplements: Hype Or Hope?

Did you know that revenue for the vitamin and supplement industry was projected to be $32 billion in 2019? And did you know that this industry is *completely unregulated*?

For anyone with health issues or vitamin/mineral deficiencies (which you can assess with a blood workup), supplementation as prescribed by a qualified medical practitioner can be extremely beneficial. But for most healthy people, study after study suggests that supplements do absolutely nothing.

The supplement industry tells us that swallowing a handful of different pills every day is in our best interest, because they can. Manufacturers are not held to any scientific standards for research whatsoever, and they can make outrageous and untrue claims as a sales hook. Everyone is wary of the greed emanating from certain pharmaceutical companies, but at least prescription medications must go through research and development, trials, and years of testing. There is a huge regulatory trail and difficult protocols to follow that lead to medications being approved. In the supplement industry, there is *nada*, and manufacturers exploit loopholes. Supplements don't fall under the label of drugs, although drug-like claims are made for them. Manufacturers use words like "could affect" or "may improve" to hoodwink their customers.

This is not to say that all supplements are bad or ineffective and that all supplement companies are scammers. But, without regulation, studies have shown that up to 40 percent of supplements tested don't even include the ingredients listed on the bottle, contain a smaller percentage of the active ingredient, and/or might well contain other ingredients they're not telling you about.

Yet I totally understand why people self-diagnose and scarf down the pills—because they don't feel listened to. Mainstream medicine does not always serve its patients well, and many people are seeking answers and looking for alternative sources because they're dissatisfied or not getting the type of attention they need from traditional sources. And, unfortunately, thanks to the lack of regulation, the supplement industry is always in your face. The options always sound so good, so promising, so *healthy*.

I have to admit that this is the only thing my wife and I argue about. She likes her supplements—I throw them out. And as for vitamin gummies for kids? This form of sugar will do nothing except give them cavities. It also teaches kids that they can get nutrients in the form of candy. Or in drink form, like Vitamin-water. Are we all really that gullible?

Please do not self-treat or think that just because something is in a bottle with a nice label, it's a safe alternative to medicine. You have *no* way of assessing its safety. You also might not know that many supplements not only have side effects on their own, but are contraindicated for those on certain prescription medications. Because supplements can often act like drugs and, therefore, interact with other drugs.

Turmeric, for example, is a well-known anti-inflammatory, but it is almost as potent as aspirin as a blood thinner that can cause you to bleed out during surgery. Melatonin is a sleep-regulating hormone that can have serious implications for your hormonal balance. DHEAS (dehydroepiandrosterone sulfate) is available over the counter but it's pre-testosterone and can lead to sex-hormone imbalances. Grapefruit juice or supplements, for example, can decrease how well your liver metabolizes certain drugs, which can then alter the drug levels in your bloodstream. Many "natural" dietary supplements have caused problems like stroke and even death.

Don't get me started on unregulated IV drips for supplementation. People are clamoring for high doses of vitamins and minerals while blithely assuming there can't be any side effects. IV drips are frequently offered without any medical supervision—by a nurse or a doctor—yet they're going directly into your bloodstream. And the colonic industry often tries to convince people that their colons are lined with the remnants of a peanut butter sandwich they ate in seventh grade. Trust me—they're not!

There are people who have true nutrient deficiencies or dietary and health restrictions who can benefit from supplements. Most experts, including the two you will hear from shortly, agree this is a case-by-case scenario. Vitamin B12 may be a good idea for vegans. Iron supplements are needed for anemic patients. Folic acid is recommended to prevent birth defects in pregnant women, and calcium and vitamin D supplements may be recommended for people at high risk for bone fractures. My general recommendation is not to take any supplement without talking to a doctor or nutritional expert first. If you think it's important enough to seek a professional's help before taking a prescription medicine, then you should be just as apt to seek professional help if you're going to be taking an unregulated supplement.

> *Healthy people eating healthy food do not need high doses of vitamins and minerals.*

Healthy people eating healthy food do not need high doses of vitamins and minerals. For me, it's much more important to focus on balance and optimization, without adding something to our daily routine. The less I put in my body, the better. I focus on good eating, good exercise, deep sleep, and daily meditation. If something goes wrong, I'll do my research, seek expert advice, and then strategize about all my options.

Stay Away from Processed Foods

When processed foods and the microwave oven came out, they were supposed to save us time and allow us to eat a better, more varied diet. If only! What have convenience foods done for our lives? They've gotten us fatter; they've taken us away from the pleasurable community of cooking together; and they've made it much harder to know what goes into our food.

You should read the labels on all packaged or processed foods. If the first few ingredients are sugar (or high fructose corn syrup) and wheat or rice flour (even if it's unbleached and/or vitamin-fortified), followed by artificial flavoring and coloring, you might want to rethink your purchase.

Take ramen. It's cheap and ubiquitous, made of pre-fried dried noodles loaded with saturated fat. The "spice" packet is basically a super-high dose of sodium, MSG, and artificial flavors. Real ramen, on the other hand, is made from bones simmered for days, so all of the nutrients and collagen become part of the delicious bone broth. Packaged ramen is a fake food and fresh ramen is a real food. Or take oatmeal. Steel-cut oats are full of fiber and extremely nutritious, but quick oats in a packet have been processed and sweetened into junk.

That doesn't mean all packaged foods are terrible. Canned tomatoes are "processed," but they're still just tomatoes and the basis for a healthy sauce. Canned tuna and salmon are "processed" too, as are frozen vegetables. The best thing to do is look for single-ingredient items, as the only processing they'll have is what was needed to can or freeze them.

Everyone wants to blame the food industry for the ready availability of junk food. People assume these companies are plotting to kill us with super-sized bottles of soda and bags of potato chips—but they're only giving the public what it wants. If there were no demand for Doritos, there would be no Doritos. Why would you expect the food business to do anything other than try to make money? You need to be wary about food-industry claims and what they're selling—but it's up to you to do due diligence about the food you buy, just as you should do due diligence before choosing a healthcare provider.

If you have questions and know you have issues with how much you're eating, it might be a good idea to seek out a qualified nutritionist for advice. There are a lot of wellness gurus out there, but many don't have degrees or experience, and they often don't have a clue what they're talking about. Some of these so-called experts are influencers on Instagram with no training whatsoever, but because they have fit and trim bodies, people pay attention. Competent advice about food is as necessary for your well-being as competent advice about your health.

Bottom line: you will generally know what and how much you're eating when you cook your own food. Restaurants and takeout establishments are in the flavor business, and they like return customers—which doesn't always align with your nutritional interests. For me, cooking is a form of meditation, and something I can do with my family. I think that's why the kitchen is always the homiest room in the house. I love to eat with other people—it goes back to that sense of community. I always eat more slowly and savor my meals when I'm with my family or friends, which is better not just for my digestion, but for my *joie de vivre*!

Food, Skin Food, and Longevity

What you eat has a direct effect on your sense of well-being and longevity—and your skin. But consuming an enormous amount of blueberries or celery juice or other items you think are "super" is not the way to deal with food. I asked Tanya Zuckerbrot, MS, RD, and the author of *The F-Factor Diet: Discover the Secret to Permanent Weight Loss*, for advice. She is a registered dietitian in private practice in New York and the founder of F-Factor, a program for weight loss and optimal health based on fiber-rich nutrition. Tanya's scientific approach to nutrition and focus on lifestyle eating habits have made her program immensely popular among many of my patients and the pro-aging lifestyle we all try to achieve.

Thinking About Pro-Aging and Healthy Eating

A Q&A with Tanya Zuckerbrot, registered dietician and author of The F-Factor Diet.

How, specifically, does food affect our skin?

As the largest organ in the body, skin needs to be nourished, just as our heart, liver, and kidneys do. A balanced diet lends itself to a healthy, clear complexion, while a poor diet can result in wrinkles, acne, and dull, dry skin. As you know, extrinsic skin aging comes from things like the sun, smoke, pollution, and poor diet. These external factors cause oxidative stress, which is the degeneration of cells and tissues and can cause signs of aging. To slow down the aging process, it is important to reduce pro-inflammatory foods and increase antioxidant- and vitamin-rich foods.

What are your top tips for improving health and longevity with how and what you eat? Are recommendations different for different people, or is it one size fits all?

There will be different recommendations for different people, but my most basic tips for improving health and longevity apply to everyone:

- *Get at least 35 grams of fiber in your diet each day.* Everyone can benefit from this. That's because fiber is the secret to permanent weight loss and management without hunger. Fiber is the indigestible part of a carbohydrate that adds bulk to food. When you follow a diet rich in fiber, you feel full after eating, so you'll generally eat less throughout the day. Also, fiber swells in the stomach, absorbs and removes fat and calories, and boosts metabolism. The average American eats less than 15 grams of fiber per day. Women need 35 grams of fiber daily, and men should aim for 38 grams.

The average American eats less than 15 grams of fiber per day. Women need 35 grams of fiber daily, and men should aim for 38 grams.

- *Drink water.* Water plays a key role in nearly every bodily function, fills you up so you tend to eat less, and helps your kidneys to rid the body of toxins and chemicals that may be slowing your metabolism. Fiber needs water to work its magic. Being dehydrated can also mimic hunger. Your body retains water when you don't give it enough. Aim for three liters of water each day to flush out your system and keep you feeling your best.

- *Focus on gratitude.* A more positive outlook can help you better manage stress, which can help decrease levels of cortisol, the stress hormone that contributes to weight gain.

What are the best foods to eat for your skin?

- *Anti-inflammatory foods* such as fruits, vegetables, legumes, and omega-3 fatty acids contain the vitamins, antioxidants, and fiber necessary to slow skin aging by minimizing degenerative effects of free radicals and oxidative stress. High-fiber foods also help flush out toxins.

- *Antioxidants* include lycopene, glutathione, flavonoids, and beta carotene (provitamin A) and can be found in carrots, tomatoes, and cocoa.

- *Sulfur-rich foods* help the body to increase production of glutathione, a powerful antioxidant. These foods include vegetables such as broccoli, brussels sprouts, and cauliflower.

- *Vitamin C* is an integral part of collagen production and is found in citrus fruits and red and yellow bell peppers.

- *Omega-3 fatty acids* help to reduce inflammation. Fatty fish is its best source for Omega-3, as it is vitamin E, a potent antioxidant that can promote skin healing.

- *Fruits and vegetables* are high in water content, and hydration is hugely important for skin health. Just like all other tissues in the body, skin cells must be adequately hydrated. Dull, dry skin, as well as skin lacking tone and elasticity, are common symptoms of dehydration.

Are certain foods pro-inflammatory and especially bad for your skin?

Yes. When fats reach the temperatures required for frying, they can oxidize, producing those free radicals that can accelerate breakdown of skin cells. Pro-inflammatory foods include:

- Fried foods
- Sugary foods
- Refined carbohydrates such as white bread, white rice, pasta
- Fruit juice
- Baked goods

What are the best choices for snacks?

A good afternoon snack is between 200–300 calories and contains at least five grams of fiber and five grams of protein.

Clinical evidence shows that fiber and protein have a high satiety benefit in calorie-controlled diets and weight reduction. The combination of fiber and protein keeps you feeling full, for the longest period of time, on the fewest calories. The fuller you feel after a meal, the less likely you'll be to overeat at the next meal and, therefore, the more likely you'll be to lose weight. Great snacks in this category include nonfat Greek yogurt and berries, jerky, or turkey pepperoni. Popcorn is low in calories and high in fiber for a delicious and satisfying snack.

Do diets ever work? Is it more important to shift your thinking away from weight loss and toward health/longevity?

If you think of a diet as a pattern of healthy eating, rather than a short-term solution to effect weight loss, then, yes, diets work. What is required is a shift in thinking. If you are focusing on health and longevity, weight is a component, and weight loss is often a welcome byproduct of getting healthier.

What is the biggest mistake people make when they want to eat better?

The biggest mistake is to cut carbohydrates, thinking this will help you lose weight. Carbs fuel our bodies, and cutting them out leads to you feeling tired, cranky, and weak. This can trigger excess snacking and feeling deprived—which is not consistent with weight loss. Cutting out carbs is also an issue because fiber, the most important tool for weight loss, is only found in carbs. They also contain essential vitamins and nutrients.

Still, while eating carbohydrates is essential to functioning, eating them in excess does lead to weight gain. The goal is to eat just the right amount of the right carbs—and this means 25–35 grams of high-fiber carbs per day.

If you have issues with food, how can you shift your thinking to make healthier choices?

The best way to shift your thinking is through education. When people understand *why* they are doing something and *how* their bodies work, they become empowered to make decisions that honor their intentions to look and feel their best. As a registered dietitian, my job is to break down the science and put it into layman's terms, so that it is more digestible and easily understandable, and disseminate it to the masses. It is then my responsibility to use my platform to share sound science, rather than my own opinions, so that my followers can make informed decisions that set them up for success for life, rather than succumb to diet fads and the ebbs and flows of wellness trends.

It's Not Just *When* You Eat, but *Why* You Eat

As a frequent referral source for my patients, I was also fortunate to speak with Dana James, MS, CNS, CDN, an expert in functional nutrition and author of *The Archetype Diet: Reclaim Your Self-Worth and Change the Shape of Your Body*. She looks at food in a unique way—combining nutritional information and science while working toward understanding the emotional component behind eating and overeating. So many of my patients come in frustrated with their relationship with food. As expected, they are looking for a procedure to speed up their progress or give them a jump start. As our self-perception seems to direct so many of our behaviors, especially eating, Dana's contribution to the pro-aging philosophy is essential.

Dealing with the Emotions of Eating

A Q&A with Dana James, nutritionist, functional medicine practitioner, and author of The Archetype Diet.

What causes people to have problems with their weight?

In my work, the fat-loss equation is food, exercise, microbiome, inflammation, hormones, and emotional suppression. The emotional component is often the missing aspect because all the other pieces are tangible, and emotions are not tangible. I use body fat as my tool to determine what is going on at a psychological and hormonal level. When I see somebody look into their childhood and release some of the trauma attached to that, their weight will drop. It doesn't matter whether they're ten or twenty or fifty pounds overweight—they'll drop five pounds. This is often missed in the sustainable weight-loss equation.

You need a harmonious lifestyle. The research on long-term weight loss shows that the best response is a combination of cognitive behavioral therapy and diet. Studies at the Rudd Center for Food Policy & Obesity at Yale showed that 76 percent of people would go to food in a stressful situation. When that happens, either adrenaline charges in and it shuts down the appetite, or cortisol makes you want to eat more, especially carbs and comfort foods that create guilt and perpetuate the cycle.

Stress-reduction techniques that work are meditation, controlled breathing, exercise, and getting into the sunshine. Making sure that you're around people who support you, feeling connected, sex—all of these reduce stress hormones. You can either sit in your stress, which is much more damaging, or you can try to find a way *not* to fall into that wound.

You can break that entire cycle by forgiving yourself and admitting, "Okay, I overeat. Let me figure out *why*." You learn from that and start to make changes. What we get upset about is not that we ate the bad food—we get upset because we're out of alignment with our integrity.

What specific foods have the greatest effect on your skin?

It's not so much a specific food as the environment of the food—the balance of what you're eating. You can eat as many blueberries or as much wild salmon as you want, but if they're paired with junk food, ice cream, and fries, and that's happening three to four days a week, you're not going to get the benefit of eating the wild salmon.

Skin, like any other organ of the body, is simply looking for an abundance of phytonutrients and antioxidants, so that you are protecting your cells from damage.

You also need fats. The Omega-6 fats (found in seeds like pumpkin, sunflower, hemp, and flax) are as necessary as the Omega-3s (found in wild salmon and fatty fish), as well as the whole spectrum of saturated fats because the cell membrane contains all of those.

Why is it so important to eat a varied diet—and not just for the nutrients?

I have many clients who eat *only* a dozen gluten-free and dairy-free foods because they think it's really healthy. They might be eating almonds every day, but then their body develops a sensitivity because they're stressed...and the stress creates gut absorption issues...then it's producing inflammation, which uses up their serotonin, which is primarily produced in the gut...and then they get depressed.

This turns into an unfortunate cycle because these people feel vulnerable and they can't figure it out because they're eating what they believe is a healthy diet. Their issue is that they're eating very few types of foods just like the standard American diet of potatoes, beef, and white flour. Variety is essential. The more colorful your food is, the better it is for you, thanks to the diversity of its nutrients.

The more colorful your food is, the better it is for you, thanks to the diversity of its nutrients.

Are there really "superfoods"?

How do we know that that a particular food has "super" nutrients? We don't; it just contains a higher dose of a particular nutrient. Brazil nuts are the highest dietary source of selenium, which supports antioxidants, but when you overdo eating them, there can be a very limited level of toxicity. We have to move away from the black-and-white thinking that "these are the *best*" and into more of the gray. And thinking more about harmony. All real foods have beneficial nutrients. It's not focusing on the best food, but getting the variety in.

What is the best way to deal with portion control?

For a woman, you're looking at half a plate of vegetables at lunch and dinner. That should be your base. And not just green veggies either. Many women who are very busy don't want to think about food, so they eat the same salad every single day. I advise them to have their salads but mix up the type of greens each day and throw in some color for variety.

One-quarter of the plate is clean protein. The remainder is split between carbohydrates or fats, depending on your goal. The fats could be olive oil as part of a dressing, a quarter of an avocado, pumpkin seeds, pine nuts, or hemp seeds.

What about the notion of "cheating"?

My rule is: once a week, have what you want. If you want to have ice cream or pasta, have it. It's going to feel good and you won't feel like you're depriving yourself. We look at flour-based products as not ideal for the skin, but in the right environment when you have all of your other antioxidants, there's nothing wrong with Dr. Frank's philosophy of "Don't cheat—treat."

"Don't cheat—treat."

The carbohydrate piece is the most controversial because we've gotten to the state that all carbs are bad, thanks to the paleo and ketogenic diets, and we need to move away from that. If you are very sensitive to carbohydrates and, when you eat them, your body very quickly puts on fat, then it might warrant you pulling them out—but that's not the vast majority of the population. Most people can handle some type of carbohydrate, such as a little bit of sweet potato, lentils, or chickpeas in the meal to make it feel more complete.

If weight loss is a goal, then keep carbs to about a quarter of a cup. The more you exercise, the more carbs you need. Otherwise, you will quickly become depleted.

How can we get the support we need—and deserve?

We need to stop denigrating women who want to look more beautiful, whether through cosmetic procedures or by losing weight. It's fascinating that, if a man says, "I've got a dad body and I want to lose weight," everyone around him is supportive. But if a woman is carrying the same amount of weight, everyone is like, "You don't need to lose weight. You're *fine*."

Why are we doing this? Are we worried that she's so fixated on her looks that she's going to become vapid? That is *not* true. If women are going to feel better or feel more confident losing the weight or doing some type of cosmetic procedure, let's support them, so they start to radiate more.

The four archetypes of women I wrote about in my book are based on where you get your self-worth from, and what I discovered is that 80 percent of women source their self-worth either from work success or family. It's those women who feel guilty about taking care of themselves. So they go on a diet for five days and then fall off. They're thinking about their weight all the time, but they're not doing anything about it because their priority is work and family, and they don't believe they're actually worthy enough to step back and take time for themselves.

If you're not getting the support you need, it's time to say, "I would really like it if you supported me, because that would mean the world to me."

CHAPTER 8

The Importance of Movement

Physical fitness is not only one of the most important
keys to a healthy body, it is the basis of dynamic
and creative intellectual activity.

—JOHN F. KENNEDY

If you try to convince people to exercise solely for its health benefits, forget it! No one's going to the gym just to improve their circulation or to get rid of high blood pressure. They're going because they want to feel and look good.

Exercise is a fantastic feedback loop because the more you move, the more you *want* to move. The number-one thing you can do for pro-aging, longevity, and beauty is to get moving. Period. Study after study after study reinforces this. Not just because it tones you, but it makes your skin brighter and it decreases wrinkles. It improves sleep and cognitive function, your immune system, and the functioning of every organ of your body—including your skin.

It's also the only thing you can do that naturally floods your body with all of the wonderful feel-good brain chemicals like dopamine and serotonin. That's why exercise is the number-one booster for mood disorders, feelings of insecurity, and emotional issues.

> *Exercise is the most effective self-empowered way to be the best version of yourself.*

Exercise is the most effective self-empowered way to be the best version of yourself. For me, the movement of my body provides as much confidence from the outside as it does on the inside.

Exercise Your Body

Nothing gives you physical and mental confidence more than exercise. But it's a process. It's hard to convince people who have never exercised that it will make them feel good if they keep at it, especially if they are overweight and ashamed or embarrassed. They might feel uncoordinated or not have a clue how to use the different machines and weights. They might not want to be around other people in a gym. But I tell them the same thing that I tell everyone: Start slowly, not only to build up stamina, but to avoid injuries. Even if you only walk for five minutes a day at first, that's great. Next week, make it ten.

Pro-Aging Tips to Bring More Movement into Your Life
Don't overdo it.
I used to go to the most intense hourlong indoor spin class four or five times a week, and, even though the workout was an intense calorie-burner, I actually gained a few pounds because I was famished afterwards. I'd eat a 2,000-calorie breakfast and still be hungry hours later. I had to find a better way—and that meant less is more.

Studies show that you need only thirty minutes of movement that elevates your heart rate, four times a week. You don't always have to work out for thirty minutes at a time—you can break it up into easily manageable segments. What's key, especially as you get older, is that, no matter how you move, you never want to do the same activity multiple times in a row. I like to alternate between aerobics one day, then strength training, then flexibility. I also like to vary my aerobics, switching between swimming, elliptical machines, and spin class, which allows me to connect to a community and encourages me to keep going.

Although modern society has become more exercise-conscious over the past couple of generations, we are also injuring ourselves more. Humans are great at assuming that if some is good, more is better—with everything. As with all medicines, there is a therapeutic window to exercise as well—a sweet spot—where we get optimum health benefits for the effort we put in. Pushing yourself well beyond this window does not correlate with an equally exponential level of improvement. But it often leads to injury or just plain physical and mental exhaustion. Obviously, this sweet spot varies due to age, genetic factors, and history of athleticism, among other factors.

I get up some days and I'm just not feeling *on*. Instead of an aerobic workout, I'll stretch, walk down from our sixth-floor apartment, and then walk the mile to work instead of going to the gym. If I do wake up and have the energy, I'll go to the gym and do a tough workout, but then I won't walk to the office.

Listen to your body. Get some form of movement in, but it doesn't have to be sweat-inducing on your low-energy days. If you're on a treadmill, for example, walk rather than run. (By the way, it's a waste of time and energy to look at the calorie counter. Yes, you will burn calories, but, more important, your metabolic rate will continue to be elevated after exercise, and that's what helps you control weight.)

Even if you can't do a dedicated exercise session, you should always move as much as you can in your daily routine.

Nothing is better than walking up and down flights of stairs instead of taking the elevator or walking on the beach or with the dog. A lot of my patients tell me about the fancy exercise equipment they buy (and then rarely use), while I know that the best athletes will tell you that all you really need are your hands and feet and a floor and gravity. Fitness is about effort, not equipment.

You don't have to join a gym—go online instead and work out at home.

One of the most beneficial ways to use the internet and streaming services is by accessing one or several of the astonishing number of videos, apps, subscriptions, and websites available for any possible kind of physical activity. The prices are low (or free) and the options are high—and getting better all the time. You can find a really good instructor who will walk you through a routine, whether it's three minutes, thirty minutes, or three hundred.

This 24/7 access has removed all excuses from finding the time to leave the house for your exercise. Even if there's a blizzard outside or you can't afford a gym, if you have a yoga mat, you can do a safe and effective workout in your home, at your convenience, with experienced instructors and all the encouragement you need.

Change up your workout as you get older.

I wish this weren't true, but as we get older, it gets harder to see and feel the results from the same exercise routines. I didn't exercise that much in college because I didn't need to. I was able to go to the gym, lift some weights, do some cardiovascular exercise to get my blood pumping, and look pretty good without thinking about it. I took my easy fitness and buff muscles for granted. Now, my metabolism has started to slow, which happens to everyone eventually, no matter how fit they are. When I go to spin classes, I would die if I tried to keep up with some of the twenty-year-olds on the bikes next to me. So I've had to completely rethink how and when I move to get the same benefits.

Don't tell yourself you can't do it.

I've had many patients tell me that they're not sporty or coordinated, and that they've never found a sport they were good at—and they're convinced they never *will* be good at it. I know this isn't true, but it's a concept that still stops a lot of people from wanting to work out.

You don't have to be good at whatever kind of exercise you do—you just have to be able to do it and be *engaged* while doing it. I was not an athlete when I was young. Until roller skating and the high school wrestling team, my greatest physical activity was watching *Gilligan's Island, The Brady Bunch*, and *I Love Lucy*! Far more crucial is the discipline it takes to get out of a warm and comfy bed to get a move on early in the morning, or to get that move on after a tiring day at work. That's the achievement.

There are tricks, but there are no shortcuts.

I tell my patients that I cannot give them advice about exercising until they empower themselves. That's true of everything—especially pro-aging. There are tricks, but there are no shortcuts. I refer my patients to classes or trainers or nutritionists (if they need to lose weight) because I'm not an expert, and they need expert advice for the next step. I have to be blunt because a large number of sedentary people come to me thinking that I can do something that will fix their problem, and that's not the case. I remind them that I bring the refinements—the icing on the cake.

Love how you exercise.
You should never force yourself to do some form of exercise you
don't really like just because you think it is good for you, and you
should never do any kind of exercise or sport that causes pain.
Exercise should never hurt. You should never be encouraged to
push yourself to the point of pain—all you'll do is get injured and
unhappy, and then you'll be out for a few months, and the whole
cycle will start over again as you try to get back into shape, physically and mentally.

I like to stretch, meditate, and do mat work. But I don't do
yoga. I forced myself to take countless yoga classes over the years
because I thought it was good for me and because I thought it
was cool. The end result: yoga was *not* good for *me*! I don't like it,
and I have an inherent inflexibility that, despite every instructor's
intent to prove me wrong, yoga just isn't my bag. When I stretch,
I prefer to be by myself or one-on-one. I know my limits. I also
know that you'll never get the best possible results from exercise
if your heart isn't in it.

For some people (like me), becoming part of a community
makes working out a whole lot more fun, and that means you're
less likely to miss your sessions. What I love about my spin class
is that I can be in the room with some hotshot twenty-year-old on
one side and a seventy-year-old grandmother on the other, and
we're all going at our own pace and working toward our own goals.
Everyone walks out with their version of a good workout that is
appropriate for their age, but with the same level of endorphin
boost. It's as much a mood booster that helps you concentrate and
focus during class and afterward as it is a physical booster that
gets your body strong. It's an active, moving meditation.

So if you don't love running on a treadmill, don't do it. If you
don't like going to a gym, don't do it. Find classes at a studio or
do workouts at home instead. There is something for everyone—
especially you!

Don't think of exercise as a chore; think of it as a challenge. You are simply challenging yourself to make improvements.

Don't think of exercise as a chore; think of it as a challenge. You are simply challenging yourself to make improvements.

It's not a pain thing. It's a not competition thing. It's just you, your body, your discipline, and your sense of empowerment.

When you hit the wall, a consultation might be helpful.
Over time, gravity pulls you down. The only thing that fights the inevitable is weight control and exercise, and, sometimes, a little professional help. A very athletic fifty-year-old who watches their weight will still see changes happening, usually with a few stubborn pounds gained that won't go away, or more fat in the abdominal area, despite copious core-strengthening exercises. This is frustrating for a lot of people, which is why they sometimes turn to treatments that might not work and could be harmful, like excessive cosmetic surgery, hormone-replacement therapy, illegal drugs, or manipulations of legal drugs. They just can't stop comparing themselves to how they were when they were younger.

Fortunately, there are many treatments and technologies that can be done now to help when people hit the wall. Over 50 percent of the work I do now is for the body in the form of scar removal, fat removal, muscle tone and development treatments, skin tightening, and fillers to shape the buttocks and deal with cellulite. The technologies I have can make safe changes in volume, shape, texture, and tone of the body, but only for those who are already in decent physical shape, who work out regularly, and who eat a healthy diet. They know that exercising doesn't make you lose weight; it helps you lose weight when you're watching what you eat. My treatments are not for weight loss.

Why Strength Training Is So Important as You Age

Longevity research continues to show that as you get older, weight lifting is just as important, if not more so, than aerobic exercise to strengthen your cardiovascular system. We lose muscle strength and mass as we get older (at least 1 percent a year after age forty), and these muscles are what support bone growth, posture, and metabolism. Muscle mass supports all aspects of our physical being, including the micronutrient levels in our body, as well as our immune system. It provides resilience and protection to our aging bodies.

It's tough as you get older to build muscle mass. One of the problems with less muscle mass is how it affects our posture. Weaker muscles mean it's harder to stand or sit perfectly upright. This becomes a vicious cycle: Thanks to muscle and bone degradation, we do less. And the less we do, the more degradation there is. The solution to this is exercise, especially weight-bearing, with either hand weights or machines in the gym, at least several times a week. The more we exercise, the more bone and muscle development there is. Strength training will be an enormous help to not only rev up your metabolism, but to improve all aspects of your movement and overall well-being.

The Profound Impact of Exercise

A Q&A with Stacey Griffith, senior master instructor at SoulCycle and motivational speaker.

Stacey Griffith has been working in the fitness industry for decades and is one of the most engaging and inspiring people I know, and she is a close friend. Her challenging physical directions, strategically choreographed set lists, and shouted-out mantras leave you on a physical and emotional high that makes you want to do more for yourself. She exemplifies pro-aging.

How does movement affect your self-image and confidence level?

Imagine for a minute that you're walking into a job interview. As you walk through the door of the building, one of the first places you feel your confidence is in your gut. When you don't feel good in the middle, it's hard to feel good anywhere else, right? That said, the way you move your body is largely determined by the current state of how you feel physically. The lighter you feel, the more confident you are.

It is not about skinny, it is not even about "super fit"—it's about feeling *light*. We move and navigate better on this planet when the insides of our bodies are operating in "light mode." My classes are always centered around riding with a light frame of mind, with a light, strong, and consistent pedal stroke. When it comes to self-image, you will *always* have a positive experience in your life if you feel a lightness in your body.

How does movement affect your skin and circulation?

I only know life in a constant state of motion. I came out of the womb swinging a tennis racket, so I know no other way than to stay in motion. This is not the average view or approach to life; some people really struggle with it. As a result of that behavior, however, I have amazing skin and fantastic circulation throughout my body...but I *earned* that.

Remember that you get out of life what you put in to it, so you have to pay your physical karmic debt in order to reap the benefits of great skin and good circulation. My philosophy is keep moving, every damn day. There are no complete days off ever—we are always moving—just some days that involve lots more rest than others. But we are *always* in motion until our number is up.

What is the emotional impact/empowerment of movement?

The amount of energy, tenacity, drive, and passion you get when you exercise is truly one of the best things about participating in it. Exercise increases levels of serotonin and dopamine in the bloodstream that keep you in a constant state of positivity. Why would you ever want to feel any other way than amazing?

Of course, life and its obstacles are always going to be there, but being in shape gives you the energy to climb the mountain rather than be tackled by the emotional negativity of the avalanche of inactivity. Don't get crushed by stagnation—get moving!

What is the minimum amount of exercise you should try to do every day? Especially as you get older?

The older you get, the more time you need to get your exercise jam on. When you're younger, you may have more energy but less time. I think it's important to balance it out and not obsess over it—there are so many variables to how much is too much. Just make sure you move every day and focus more on how healthy you eat *first*; focus on exercise second. Eating healthy is the number-one way to guarantee health.

How can you incorporate regular movement into your daily routine?

Find a way to walk more. It is that simple. Walking is such a sneak-attack way to burn calories and increase blood flow. Take the stairs more and skip a step while flexing your booty, and walk slower up the stairs in a more concentrated way. You will be shocked at how tight your ass feels by the end of the day. It is literally one of the best ways to keep your body toned. *Walk!*

If your energy flags, what are some tips to rev it back up?

We all need to hydrate more with water. Drink water all day long and you won't be tired if you watch how many sugars and carbs you put in your mouth. Stay on a balanced diet and you won't crash. Sugar, caffeine, and carbs steal your energy.

What kind of excuses have you heard from people who know they should move more but just don't? How do you get them motivated?

Depression is the motivation thief. The more you move, the more chances you have at running past depression. Exercise is the number-one prescribed medicine for depression, and I always say you gotta move to lose the blues. Go for a run, a bike ride, or take a class that has action-based movements, dynamic instructors, and a good tribe of people, and you will crush your life!

If you aren't yet as in shape as you want to be, how can you turn off the negativity/self-doubt and empower yourself to develop a healthy body image?

You have to stop comparing yourself to the world. This is your life, your experience, your journey. The image of who you are has taken a long time to come together, and it will always be morphing, growing, and building. For each mistake we make in life, we add another good story. I think this is a *perfect* thing to remember about self-love.

We need experiences to make up who we are as humans. If you are in a rut, a dip, a hole, a canyon, it's time for you to climb out. If you find it hard, struggle back out and stand up for yourself by asking someone fit for help. As a fit person, it always makes me *so* happy when someone asks me for help. Remember, none of us do it alone, and none of us is ever alone. We do it *together*.

CHAPTER 9

Managing Your Stress and Sleep

To be yourself in a world that is constantly trying to make you something else is the greatest accomplishment.

—RALPH WALDO EMERSON

Stress, like the toxins in our environment, is unavoidable. Managing your stress is at the very heart of pro-aging: by giving yourself the time you need for sleep and for finding a way to calm your brain and body for the challenges of daily life.

Stress is normal and can even be beneficial at times, but controlling it makes all the difference. How do you do that? By giving yourself the appropriate time to repair and refresh. Anything you do to strengthen and improve your body makes you look good as well. As aggressive as it might seem when you do things like laser resurfacing, you're actually recharging and repairing your skin by getting rid of the old and stimulating the new.

It's the same with sleep and meditation—the two most useful stress-busters I know. Meditation isn't some magic medicine.

Like a restful night in slumber, it's allowing the amazing machine that is your body to get rid of the built-up psychological and physiological crap you accumulated during the day, so your cells and organs can function efficiently. Most of what you can do to live a better-looking and better-feeling life is merely giving your body the opportunity to do its job.

What Stress Does to Your Skin

How Does Stress Affect the Skin?

When your body is challenged, your stress hormones kick in so you can try to manage the situation. The two main ones are cortisol and adrenaline, primarily released by the adrenal glands. These stress hormones help regulate your immune system, your metabolism, the rest of your hormones, cellular activity, and just about every other function of the body. Not having enough of these natural chemicals can have a detrimental effect, just as having too much of them can. Disease states where they are in excess or depletion can wreak havoc on the body. Stress and challenge, to some degree, are an essential part of our evolution and well-being. Balance is key as with all things pro-aging.

Stress and the hormonal symphony as a whole affect the aging process, the look of your skin, and the ability for your everyday functions to work for you or against you. If you're wondering why you can't lose weight, have trouble building muscle mass, have sleep irregularities, irregular periods, dark circles under your eyes, skin issues such as acne, and/or sexual dysfunction...think about stress and the physiologic changes that go along with it. It's easier said than done to "manage your stress," but these facts certainly make it a priority.

Now I don't believe that stress is the origin of all medical maladies, including the ones in the previous paragraph, but there is no question in my mind that stress is a huge exacerbating factor. People ask me if stress causes their acne or eczema. Believe it or not, it was believed by doctors years ago that many such skin diseases were a direct result of neurosis. My answer is always the same: if stress were the root cause of any disease, we would all be dead by now...with pimples. It would be great to have such a simple response, but, yes, some vacation time, a good night's sleep, and falling in love, among other stress-reducing activities, certainly help most chronic medical issues of any kind. So be aware of what is stressing you out and try to figure out ways to control it.

One of the main issues of modern-day life is not just the physiologic change of stress itself, but the endless abuse of the medications and intoxicants people turn to in order to manage the stress. Pharmaceutical management of stress is a multibillion-dollar business, legal and illegal. Have you ever needed to "take the edge off"? You're not alone, legal or illegal, there will always be someone out there offering and selling a means to do so. Antidepressants, anti-anxiety meds, sleeping pills, opioid medications, weight-loss drugs, brain-focusing stimulants, and every other drug cocktail are what people use as they try to manage the side effects of the cumulative physiologic changes of "stress" and the conditions associated with it. An enormous percentage of the pharmaceutical industry profits come from treating "side effects" of stress without worrying about the side effects these medicines themselves will cause, including dependency. They have more drugs to sell to help with that too, which is exactly why most people aren't taking just one medicine. The list goes on and on. Are any of these chemical answers working to fix the actual cause of these problems?

As a doctor, I believe all these agents have a role in the practice of medicine. It is not within the scope of this book to help decide who needs them or not. What I want to do is have the conversation—to get my patients and to get you to think about these issues. It is the first step toward finding balance. We live life once. There is nothing wrong with altering our senses for recreation and using modern medicine to help manage our health while interacting with the world we live in, as long as it doesn't have an abusive effect on ourselves and those around us. Everything we put into our body has a cost/benefit ratio. Certainly, there is a problem, though, with society's relationship with intoxicants and medications. And the solution to any mass problem of a population starts with the thinking of a single individual. The costs eventually outweigh the benefits when we ignore the root of the problem and the behaviors that cause them.

Try to Get Enough Sleep

There's no way you can ever manage your stress quickly and well—or look your best—if you're exhausted from a lack of sleep. It's called *beauty sleep* for a reason!

When was the last time you got enough sleep so that you woke up feeling fantastically refreshed? Was it back when you were a teenager and could sleep for thirteen hours straight? The most common complaint my patients have is they can conk out easily, but then wake up way too early and can't fall back asleep.

I know how they feel, because it happens to me all the time. Maybe I have to pee. Maybe the dog barked. Maybe my brain just told me I forgot to return that email I promised to send. But the end result of not getting enough sleep over a period of time is a genuine health hazard.

Sleep is a complicated physiologic action, regulated by the two hormones, melatonin and cortisol, that manage your circadian rhythm. As evening arrives, melatonin levels rise to make you sleepy, and then, before dawn, normal levels of cortisol kick in to help get you up. The function of sleep is a regulatory mechanism for recovery and repair for all the functions of your body, both physical and mental. These repair functions are optimized at this time because you're not in a state where you're constantly challenging them.

Most adults need between seven to nine hours of sleep every night—and they need it consistently. You can't be sleep-deprived from Monday to Friday and then think you can make it up on weekends. Don't be impressed with anyone who says they are good on only four hours of sleep a night. They are not!

However, the need for sound sleep does decrease as you get older, and we tend to sleep for shorter stints of time and perhaps feel less rested.

The biological repercussions of sleep deprivation are alarming. Chronic sleep deprivation affects your immune system resulting in more colds or flu. It can make you depressed and anxious as it affects memory and organized thought processes. It can increase risk of heart attack, stroke, high blood pressure, and a lower libido in addition to weight gain, as sleep helps regulate your metabolism and the use of food energy.

No wonder you feel so awful when you don't get enough sleep. Your body is telling you something.

Wind Down Before Bedtime

There are countless books, apps, articles, and doctors all trying to help people sleep. No one has come up with a universal solution, but these tips have helped me on sleepless nights:

- Look at your daytime activities. Meditation and exercise are the best ways to maximize your sleep, as I'll describe later in this chapter.
- Have your bedroom be a calm and peaceful environment for sleeping. The bedroom is for two main functions: sleeping and sex! Get everything else out of the room. If

you work on your computer in bed, guess what you'll be thinking about whenever you're in bed?

- Don't drink anything caffeinated or stimulating after noon, because there's always some caffeine residue circulating in your bloodstream. This is particularly hard for me, as I do love an afternoon coffee.
- Don't exercise within three hours before bedtime. Even though regular exercise is good for you and will help you sleep better, doing it too close to bedtime will rev up your entire body.
- Don't use alcohol as a sleeping aid. Convincing yourself that a drink right before you go to bed is going to give you a better night's sleep is like telling yourself that one more glass of Bordeaux is good for your heart. It's just not true. Alcohol affects your sleep cycle and sleep quality. If you drink heavily and go to sleep, your body needs to metabolize and get rid of the toxic metabolites instead of replenishing itself. You want your body to be recharged and ready for the next day, not still dealing with the after-effects of the night before.
- All electronics should be turned off and put away at least an hour before bedtime. Keep your TV and computer out of your room, if possible. One look at a problem email or energizing TV show and your brain will wake up just when you want it to slow down.
- Have a bedtime routine. If you've raised children, I'll bet you tried to create a soothing bedtime routine for your little ones: bath, bottle, book, lullaby, night-night. Why not do the same for yourself?
- It also helps to go to bed within forty-five minutes of the same time every night for at least four weeks, even if you're not fully tired. This can be an effective sleep training, no matter what your age.

- Try not to eat within two to four hours before your bedtime, as digestion takes time and energy. I know that I won't have a good, sound sleep if I have a late dinner. Many people have told me they use food as a means to get tired, as they know that they feel sleepy after a big meal. But if your body needs to expend its energy digesting your meal, it won't have as much of that energy for the recharging and refreshing processes it needs to do during sleep. And sleep is equally as important for your metabolic weight control.

  If you've had one of those days where you didn't have time to eat dinner at your normal time and you're hungry, of course you should eat something. Choose foods that are light, lack sugar or caffeine, and that digest quickly.

Try to Get a Power Nap

I love napping. As part of my twenty minutes of afternoon meditation, I often conk right out—what I like to call my "transcensnoozal napitation." I've always been lucky that way, and it certainly helped during my long hours of hospital training. Some people are nappers and others can't nap, no matter how little sleep they get.

If you're very tired and wish you could nap, you can still give yourself a short period of relaxation in a quiet room. Meditate or let your mind wander. It'll be refreshing and rejuvenating—even if you're a bit bored, then you're achieving something. My goal now is to have that time to be bored!

Avoid All OTC or Prescription Sleep "Aids"

We live in a culture where sleep aids are sold like candy. I have a lot of patients who live on Ambien, a prescription-only hypnotic agent, which can have a lot of side effects. Like every new wonder drug, Ambien's release came with the promise of non-addiction and no side effects. Think again! Patients who chronically take it put themselves at risk for sleepwalking issues, memory loss, and, most important, dependency. Yet, when Ambien first came out, you'd never have known any of these negative side effects were possible. Sort of like how Oxycontin, SSRI (selective serotonin reuptake inhibitor) antidepressants, and Valium were initially thought of as miracle workers too. Historically, nothing changes people; only the stories change. You might not know that cocaine used to be in a well-known carbonated drink, morphine was a common ingredient in childhood cough medicines, and heroin was briefly touted as a miracle drug for most maladies at the turn of the twentieth century.

I have many other patients who self-medicate with various homeopathic, holistic, herbal, and melatonin supplements, which are readily available OTC. You can even get them in gummy form for *children*.

I don't recommend regular use of any sleep aids. If you have recurring sleep issues, you should always consult a doctor for expert advice before buying a supplement. Just because a supplement is OTC doesn't mean it's safe or effective. *All* sleeping-pill sleep is false sleep. Looking for a quick fix might help you fall asleep for a few nights, but they're only good for short-term use.

Most important, regardless of the class of pharmacology that you're using to go to sleep, sleeping pills are addictive. Not all of them are addictive *physically,* but they're often addictive *psychologically*. This in turn worsens the original problem when trying to get off them.

The One Sleep Aid that Works

The very best sleep aid doesn't cost anything. It's exercise. The more you exercise, the better you sleep. It uses up valuable energy, it helps regulate circadian rhythm, metabolism, and hormonal fluctuations.

When You Wake Up in the Middle of the Night

I almost always fall right asleep because I've worked hard all day, exercised, meditated, and eaten an early supper. I'm pooped! But my biggest sleep issue is waking up in the middle of the night and not being able to fall right back asleep.

When that used to happen, I'd get up and go to the bathroom and, within three minutes, I would know if there was going to be a falling-back-to-sleep problem. I'd get mad at myself, and then my mind would just start going...and going. I'd go back to bed and toss and turn. I was tired and stressed, even as I told myself to stop, as stress begets stress. Sometimes, I'd fall back asleep, but, most of the time, it would take a minimum of an hour for that to happen.

One of the reasons for this is because I spend my work days working frenetically taking care of other people, and I don't have the bandwidth to daydream about the important things in life outside of my job. I work instinctually and reflexively, so when I'm forced into a situation where I can't sleep, I set strict rules for myself. I get up out of bed and go into the living room—I know I need to get out of the zone of stress, which, at that moment, is the bedroom. Often, I'll meditate to clear my mind. I put effort into taking stock of the gifts in my life. I focus on the now. And then, at those moments, my stress goes away and I'm no longer worrying about my busy schedule in the morning or a patient who needed some extra care. I realize that there is absolutely nothing I can do about any of those situations at the moment, so I will instead focus on the things I have. If I'm going to think about the past, I'm going to reflect on memories of good times with my family and friends. If I'm going think about the future, it will be about those types of positive things too.

Sometimes, if I'm not in the mood to daydream or meditate, I'll read; I'll pick up a book or, more often, listen to an audio book, which I love to do because, as in childhood, who doesn't like being read a story to make you go to sleep? If I'm by a clock or my phone, forget about it. It's not easy, but I force myself not to look at it. I can't turn my phone off because I'm always on call in case of a patient emergency, but I really try not to pick it up. Since I've done that, ninety-five out of a hundred times, I end up falling asleep on the couch for the rest of the night, or I start dozing and go back to bed.

Still, I'm not always good at doing this. Some nights are going to be all about tossing and turning, no matter what. It's very easy to say, "Get out of your mind," but it can be very difficult to do that when stress is overwhelming.

But this too shall pass. When I am doing everything I can to be pro-aging—when I meditate, when I eat well, when I exercise—I find that things get better as a whole and I'm less likely to get caught up in a crappy night here and there.

This is true of everything pro-aging. Take stock of the big picture and your ultimate goals. We can't control every moment and we will never be perfect. Isn't that consoling? We are all not perfect, and never will be! My father always likes to quote Margaret Atwood: "As you ramble through life, whatever be your goal, keep your eye on the doughnut, and not on the hole."

Pro-Age Your Way to Calm with Meditation

Meditation changed my life.

With my background and training in conventional Western medicine, in my early stage of training, I used to think of meditation as nonsensical, with no grounding in science. I fully admit to being closed-minded about other healing options outside the confines of my rigorous by-the-book approach to medicine. As for beliefs of a more spiritual nature, well, I was raised by a Sicilian Roman Catholic mother and a mixed-European Jewish father. Nonetheless, religion played very little role in my upbringing. We ate a lot, laughed a lot, liked to disco roller skate, and spoke loudly and above each other most often—and that was a great formula for family in my household.

With time and experience and all the wonders of cutting-edge technology that informed my practice over the years, I came to realize that we don't know as much as we think we know. Every generation, going back to the Dark Ages, was filled with people who were oh-so-sure that they had all of the answers already. But, of course, there are limits to science, and there's so much more that we have to learn—and, often, unlearn because studies that once determined that something was healthy have since been debunked.

I think the biggest intellectual accomplishment any human being can make is admitting how little they know, even about topics they have studied or practiced in depth and are considered expert on. As the world-renowned cellist Pablo Casals famously said when asked why he continued to practice for at least four hours every day, well into his nineties: "Because I think I am making progress."

For me, the realization of how little I know caused a seismic shift in my thinking. Amusingly, my wife, Diana, was inspirational in this realization. As we get older, we often get set in our ways. People are naturally afraid of health problems and of looking old or feeling old, so there's a reflexive tendency to stick with what they know. I totally understand why people act that way—because that was me. Until I discovered the power of meditation.

Diana has always been more spiritually inclined than I, so, six years ago, I gave her an intensive training session of Transcendental Meditation (TM) as a birthday gift. I said that I would do the training with her and be open to it. This wasn't just because it was a gift she would appreciate, but, on a more selfish level, I knew something had to change in my life. I'd gotten to a point emotionally and professionally where I'd pretty much exceeded my dreams. I had a smart and beautiful wife, gorgeous and healthy kids, and a very successful practice where I was in the right place in the right time. But even with all those blessings, I was often shocked at how much frustration I allowed into my life. I felt that the more success I had, the more I was losing touch with my appreciation for it and for everyone that I took care of. Financial success brought many unexpected pressures, as well as people who invaded my life with their own toxicity. The demands of success left me with zero time in the day for all of the simple things that made me happy—like spending downtime with my family and friends, listening to music, dancing, and cooking. What was the point of having all that success, health, love, and *stuff* if I could no longer be grateful for it or appreciate it? I felt spoiled and stuck. I was on a treadmill to nowhere.

Even though I told Diana I was going into the training with an open heart and mind, I was, to be honest, not quite there yet. Funnily enough, I've been told that the people who are most type A, most driven, and most I-don't-have-time-for-this-type-of-thing are actually the most susceptible to the powers of meditation. Clearly, we need it, and I was happy to find out that once it clicks, the discipline of doing it is easier for us type-A folk—we can be a bit OCD with habits.

I was also a bit skeptical about Transcendental Meditation. I only knew that it had been developed by the Maharishi Mahesh Yogi—the guy the Beatles went to see in India during their so-called spiritual phase in the mid-1960s. (At that point, the Maharishi had already been teaching his system for over a decade.) While researching it, I learned that TM has had the highest amount of peer-reviewed scientific studies over the years—investigating its benefits for reducing high blood pressure, in drug recovery, the prison rehabilitation system, helping veterans with PTSD, and with several types of chronic disease. In fact, a 2012 review of 163 studies published by the American Psychological Association concluded that Transcendental Meditation helped to "reduce anxiety, negative emotions, trait anxiety, and neuroticism while aiding learning, memory, and self-realization."

The rigorousness of all these studies was the primary reason why TM appealed to me. Followed by the fact that it was nonreligious and more focused on the health and quality of life—one of the keys to pro-aging. I was still skeptical that sitting still and saying some mantras could do all that, but I had nothing to lose by trying it. And, of course, much to gain.

During the training, you are first introduced to TM as a group. Then you have a private session with your instructor, who gives you a mantra that is unique (and sacred) to you, and not to be shared. After a consecutive four-day period for about two hours a day, you're off to the races—that's it. There are "check-ins" a week or two later to address how you are doing, but, overall, it was amazingly simple. That was the point. Every person at every training center (supported by the David Lynch Foundation) around the world is trained exactly the same way. There is no additional sales pitch; instead, you have unlimited access to the resources of your local center and community. The more people that do TM, the better, calmer, clearer, and more engaged individuals they become, and the better a world community we all become for it.

Positive, fulfilled energy, like toxic energy, is contagious. Once you reap the benefits of TM, your filters and attraction to people, environment, and situations completely change. Your tolerance for things and people that drain you become less, and your recognition and attraction for things that are positive and productive become stronger. You don't change or become a different person. You literally just start feeling like a better version of yourself, which, as you can imagine, affects everything from how you feel to how you look in the mirror.

I faithfully did my twice-daily sessions and noticed something positive right away. It took a few weeks to get into the habit. I probably get in twelve of the fourteen-per-week sessions. Sometimes I don't get in the whole twenty minutes. Sometimes all I think about is work or I fall asleep. Sometimes, I am super stressed, and I wonder if it's doing anything for me anymore. But, like exercise and nutrition, whatever I do to make an effort is better than none at all. I am positive that I am a better person for it, better for myself and therefore better for others.

That's the beautiful thing about TM: there's very little wrong you can do. It works for everyone because it's about giving your brain the opportunity to do what it wants to do—chill the hell out. For me, it's having that time to let work stuff go. I'll sit on my chair in my private office, and a few head bobs later, I come back to reality and wonder, Was I asleep? Was I awake? Maybe I did nod off for a few minutes, but whatever it was, I'm just refreshed.

Ideally, I do my second session in the middle of my workday, and if that's not feasible, I try to do it as soon as I get home from work. I'll even do it while riding in a car. So when people ask me how I find the time, I ask them how they find the time to shower and blow-dry their hair, then explain that you're supposed to do your first meditation before you challenge yourself for the day. I get up and brush my teeth, get my wits about me, and then sit in a comfortable chair or on the side of the bed and do it.

If I miss more than a few sessions each week, I feel the effects right away. There are times when I miss a meditation, and I later get the feeling like I went to work forgetting to shave or brush my teeth! My meditation time is now such an ingrained part of my day and so crucial to my pro-aging well-being that I can't imagine not doing it.

If you think you don't have the time, what you'll be shocked by is how much time each day you actually waste on things, people, and repetitive thoughts that have no positive impact on your life. Instead, with your meditative practice, you are actually *gaining* time for the things life is worth living for. Just give it a shot!

Why Meditation Is Pro-Aging

Part of what makes any kind of meditation so effective is that it's a daily habit. I know some people think that they can go off on a meditation retreat for a few days and reap the benefits for many months to come. That's not how it works...just as crash diets or extreme exercise routines don't work over the long term. They're quick fixes. Meditation is a *long* fix for life. Once you incorporate such a good habit into your daily routine, it becomes effortless. It's not a chore. You look forward to it because you know how good it makes you feel. (This is how you should feel about exercise as well.) That's the *pro*gressive and *pro*found part of pro-aging.

What I love most about TM is how it sends me right into a kind of free-flowing state of mind that often leads to not thinking at all. This is the "zone" that is used euphemistically in everything from professional sports to the arts. It's where creativity breeds and where excellence comes from. There are times you fall asleep and times you stress about work, and there are times when you go into a sort of trance where you don't know if you are awake or asleep. If there is a goal to meditation—this is it. As soon as you come out of it, you feel as if you had taken the most refreshing nap. In fact, meditation has the same refreshing effect on your brain and body in a shorter time than a nap and is so helpful because most people don't have the option to take a nap undisturbed during the day.

Whatever form of meditation you do, one of the most satisfying benefits is that it helps you sleep better. It not only refreshes you when you do it, but it also reduces stress and anxiety, which are the two most common causes of insomnia. Intense meditation practices help to achieve a harmony between body and mind. Study after study confirms meditation practices clearly affect brain functions, from its metabolism, hormone production, neurologic pathway plasticity, and neural wave form—all of which help mediate its regulatory functions.

I also believe that meditation helps with sleep and replenishment because it clears the space for you to focus on what you value most—the people you love, and your self-care. As you get older, you have family responsibilities, a busy career, you're aging, you're dealing with the vulnerabilities of life's processes. Your personal, fine-tuned radio station develops a lot of static. Meditation is what tunes in and calibrates the radio station of your life to get rid of that static. This is what ultimately allows you to vibrate and function at a higher level. It doesn't require research data to realize this feeling has advantages for all aspects of your life.

There is no "best" meditation—only what's best for *you*. Like every other pro-aging strategy in this book, what works most effectively is that something that instinctively clicks with your personal sensibility. Remember, any effort is better than no effort, even if you can only meditate for five minutes at a time. Merely sitting in a quiet place, with no cellphones, music, or other distractions, with eyes open or shut, and letting your mind wander, is what allows the exhaust valve of life to open. It gets the gunk out.

Meditation makes you stronger, more centered, and more focused. It allows you to say, "I *need* this time now for myself." I worked as an EMT in college, and rule number one is to protect yourself first. At an accident site or in the ER, if someone has died or is clearly dying, you're no good to anybody else if you can't protect yourself first. It's the mental and emotional equivalent of pro-aging's definition of vanity: it's not wrong to think of your own needs, to lead a better, happier, more empowered life. Others around you will benefit from it as well.

Moving Meditation

TM is always done in a seated position, and this is one of the reasons why it is so calming and stress-relieving.

I also like more energizing meditations, done when you're in motion. It's ideal for stress relief, and if it's part of your exercise routine, you're maximizing your time to do two pro-aging categories at once. Here's how:

Pick a low-impact activity with repetitive simple motion you can do reflexively, like walking or swimming. Do this on your own and turn your phone off (or leave it someplace where you won't look at it). Do not talk to anyone. Do not listen to music. Focus solely on the movement itself. Make sure you are in a safe environment where you can't get hit by a car or be injured due to not paying attention to your surroundings.

The repetitive motion puts your mind and body in a more effortless state, allowing you to shift consciousness, rest, and recuperate. For me, the greatest moving meditation is walking on a beach or swimming on a hot day. The environment, the activity, the energy I get—it's like a greatest hits of pro-aging. It makes me feel good to be alive. And that's a pretty good daily goal, right?

Pro-Aging Tips for Stress Management

Stress management is about self-care. if you can't manage your own stress, you can't help other people.

In my practice, I personally see twenty-five to thirty-five patients a day, and another thirty go through my office. These patients all come for some form of self-improvement, much like others go to a spiritual leader, a personal trainer, or a nutritionist. Anyone who is in the service industry gets the opportunity to see the best and worst of the human element. I do have patients who are police officers or in the armed forces (they want to look good too!), and, like doctors, they see the best and worst of people.

When things go well, our jobs are extremely uplifting professions. But when you see the worst of people, it's very tough to stay on the sharp and narrow, remain positive, and not absorb the stress.

For me, the best stress-buster is to spend time with my family and friends. That's due to the fact that most of the things that give me stress in life are related to *myself*. The ego that relates to work. How I'm taking care of my patients. How I'm performing. Wondering whether I'm doing too much of this or not enough of that.

A lot of stress comes from fear. Your mind is a great tool, but it's by far your worst enemy.

I love getting outdoors. I love going to the beach and the mountains, looking at nature, and relishing the fact of being small. Our problems are not always enormous. We can prepare all we want for our presence and exit from this world, but the things that get you are usually not the things that you spent your whole life stressing about. We're all going to die one day, and it will probably not be from the thing we're constantly trying to avoid.

Every time I think of that, I get a craving for an Insomnia chocolate chip cookie!

Stop Blaming Yourself

Many of my patients are new mothers who are very stressed. A lot of them struggled to get pregnant, and they confide in me before and during their pregnancies, as they need to tell me if they're on any medications for fertility issues or anything else. They've had a tough time, physically and emotionally, and we talk, as I offer them options about getting rid of the hyperpigmentation spots that are common with pregnancy, or weight loss, or just helping them look less exhausted.

The most common thing they stress about is that they think they're doing everything wrong. I always tell them that, when you question yourself, it makes you a better person. If you're worrying about your baby, or your job, or any of the people in your orbit, that tells me you're actually good at what you do and that you really care. The crummy parents and business owners are the ones who don't care or self-monitor. Recognize that you are not the first to go through any challenge. It's been done before. As I said already, you're special but you are not uncommon! Communicate with people. Share your concerns. Be open-minded and don't let anyone tell you there is only one right way to do things. Most important, be kind to yourself. Adaptability is by far the most essential skill in life. As Charles Darwin purportedly said, "It is not the strongest of the species that survives, nor the most intelligent that survives. It is the one that is the most adaptable to change."

Focus on the Now

Much of our stress comes from focusing on things that happened in the past that we can't undo, or focusing on things in the future that may or may not happen, certainly not in the way we envision them. We tell ourselves that if we make more money, we can do this, or if we're better-looking, we can do that, or if we lose ten pounds, we'll find that perfect partner. Or we keep asking ourselves why we didn't do XYZ when we had the chance.

The author Eckhart Tolle famously said in *The Power of Now* that there is no past or future; there's only just now. Focusing on the right-now will help you take care of the future that hasn't happened yet. I've found that when I do that, a lot of my stress evaporates because I'm not worrying about the hypothetical what-ifs. We have to keep remembering to take things moment by moment and day by day.

When thinking about the right-now, I am often reminded that the two most common questions people ask me about my business are: "What are your hours?" and "What's your end game?"

As if I am running a grueling race, with a finish line of prizes to look forward to. I tell them that my hours are "eyes opened to eyes closed." But I don't think of it as if I'm a workaholic, because I'm passionate about and love what I do. As for my end game, well, I usually say, "I don't know...death?"

More than anything, I worry about my patients every day. They typically say, "Promise me, Doctor, that this is safe." I tell them that I promise I'm going to give my very best attention, and I'm performing something with their consent that is as safe as possible. But nothing in this world is 100 percent safe, not walking out of your house or drinking a cup of water or taking an aspirin. Anyone who tells you otherwise is lying to you. All medical procedures have risks. Sometimes things don't always go as planned, and the greatest skill that I could have as a physician is to manage the tough times. It's easy when everyone's happy and hugging me after their face shots and lasers go well. It's not easy when someone comes to me for a procedure and it turns out there's a complication—it happens.

So my end game is my right-now. If you keep thinking about what you're going to do in the future to reduce your stress, then you're not focusing on what you can do right now to deal with it. It's okay to daydream about a successful future, but I've never met anybody who had a thriving business and sold it for a lot of money and said, "You know, those daydreams I had about selling my business turned out exactly how I wanted them to." It never happens like that. My great-aunt Fran used to always say to me, "Be careful what you wish for—it just may come true."

The only thing that is limiting for all of us in life, no matter what our financial or any other situation, is our health. As a doctor, I know that it's one thing you can't buy and that you sometimes can't change. Of course, if you're sick, you can do things to take care of yourself. But, unfortunately, people get hit with lightning in the form of bad news about their health all the time, and I constantly remind myself how lucky I am because, as long as I'm here, I'm healthy and I have my faculties, I'm in good shape.

One of the titles I had for a future book was *Playing with the House's Money* because that's how to look at life. If you have your basic needs and your health, you're playing with the house's money. Many of the creative endeavors I have in business and where I'm taking my practice of medicine have come about because I view life that way. It doesn't mean I'm risking or gambling everything, but that I recognize I have my basic needs met and that I'm blessed in so many ways. If all of my lifestyle things are taken away, I'd still be in good shape; some of the most inspirational people I've ever read or met are those who do not need a lot of things. I can't tell you how many of my patients get to a certain age and realize how much time they spent acquiring things that only made their lives more complicated, and how useless those things turned out to be. They want to downsize because life is simpler that way.

With a lot less stress.

Find Your Pleasures and Enjoy Them

We all need harmless entertainment—to be taken out of our lives and stresses and to just have fun. These are "guilty pleasures." Not every activity has to be productive!

Entertainment should not make you feel guilty. Life isn't just about work. Or it shouldn't be. Your brain and body need downtime. So enjoy it!

> *Not every activity has to be productive!*

Putting Pro-Aging into Practice

> There is a fountain of youth: It is your mind,
> your talents, the creativity you bring to your life and
> the lives of the people you love. When you learn to tap
> this source, you will truly have defeated age.
>
> —SOPHIA LOREN

Pro-aging, as you know by now, is not a diet or a regimented workout. It's a transition to the rest of your life.

Not that long ago, I was talking about my fairly regimented lifestyle habits to a younger patient, when he asked how I stay looking and feeling so young. Obviously, this schedule makes me seem quite boring (I used to be much cooler in my youth)—going to bed by 10:00 p.m., not drinking any alcohol on weekdays, and generally avoiding the bread basket and French fries on the dinner table. I told him, "I know it makes me sound like an old man," but maintaining these habits makes me feel and perceive myself as younger, more energetic, and confident. When I eat and sleep irresponsibly, as I used to, and have crappy lifestyle habits associated with *young* people, that's when I feel *old*!"

Even though my workdays are very busy with seeing patients, running my business, teaching, writing, conducting research, and consulting, I always find time to connect with my family, refresh with meditation, nourish with a healthy diet, and move with morning exercise. I'll do five days of fast mimicking three times a year to give my body the break it needs, usually after vacation indulgences. Honestly, I can't recall over my fifty years ever feeling so good, so strong, so vital, and self-confident. That doesn't seem boring at all, does it?

Your body wants to nourish and care for itself. It's built to do that, when given the chance. One million years of evolution is a lot more informative and useful than an infomercial selling you "what you need." When you stay away from things that aren't good for you, even for a little while, your body repairs itself. You just need to give your body time to do what it's supposed to do. I always say to my patients, "You can't get a bruise to go away until you stop punching yourself in the arm."

The best way to incorporate all of my pro-aging advice into a lifestyle that works for you is to start slowly—one step at a time. One exercise routine, one dietary change, one product or procedure at a time until you're sure it works for you. When in doubt, follow my dad's rule of KISS.

Give yourself thirty days for a pro-aging reboot. Most experts agree that positive and negative habits can be developed or broken over thirty to ninety days. Incremental changes will end up giving you big results.

Life has stresses and endless challenges. They are essential for change and progress for all forms of life on our planet. But success in life is about balance, and pro-aging is all about finding that balance and maximizing it for optimal health and beauty. The future is bright in our ability to live longer and better lives. What is most clear is the need for us all to be active participants in our own well-being. Feeling vital won't just happen to us as we age.

To educate ourselves, to participate, and to be proactive in being the best we can be, so we can live a life of joy. The good news is that, if we are lucky, it's a long life. How we navigate it will make all the difference in how we look and feel about ourselves, how we interact with the world around us, and how much we get to enjoy the ride. The secret of life is quite simple, and it comes down to merely enjoying the passage of time.

I wish you all happy pro-aging.

ACKNOWLEDGMENTS

Thank you first and foremost to my immediate and extended family for your unrelenting love. My parents for putting me where I am today. My wife, Diana, for her nurturing and tolerance. My children, Aidan and Avery, for keeping me humble. Most important, my sister and PFRANKMD director of operations, Annie, for being so instrumental in making all my professional ideas and goals come to life. To my office family of valuable staff members, thank you for always keeping me moving and being the extra hands I do not have. Thank you to all my patients for your trust throughout the years.

I would not be where I am today without the guidance of my physician mentors and peers. Thank you for teaching me how to care for people. Drs. Rhoda and David Narins, Dr. Phillip Orbuch, and Dr. Rena Brand—thank you for giving me the opportunities and skills early in my career to make my professional dreams come true.

I could not have provided the complete picture of The Pro-Aging Playbook without the contributions of my valuable experts. Thank you, Dr. David Rosenberg, as you continue to guide me and lead by example in more ways than you know. Thank you, Dr. Michael Apa—you set the bar quite high in your meticulousness and enthusiasm for aesthetic healthcare. Thank you, Georgia Louise—your aesthetic style and complementary talents are essential to my efforts and outcomes. Christopher Drummond, your talents continue to amaze me. Thank you for all your contributions to PFRANKMD. Stacey Griffith, you are an inspiration and motivator in every aspect of my life. Thank you for your unstoppable energy. Tanya Zuckerbrot and Dana James—thank you for taking care of so many of my patients throughout the years and sharing your passion for food and life.

Thanks to Anthony Ziccardi and the people at Post Hill Press for their support, giving me creative freedom and their belief in this project. Thank you, Lauren Marino, for your organizational contributions and clarity for this book. Thank you to Kenyon and Eryn Phillips at MRMRS CREATIVE for their artistic contributions to the book and to my entire professional life. You both just get me.

To Janet Goldstein, my agent and quarterback—your opinions, feedback, handholding, and guidance during this past year are so appreciated. Thank you.

Most important, this book would not have been possible without Karen Moline, whose writing skills, friendship, and enthusiasm for this project inspired me throughout the process. No one could have translated my thoughts better than you. Thank you from the bottom of my heart.

ABOUT THE AUTHOR

Dr. Paul Jarrod Frank is one of the most influential cosmetic dermatologists in the world. Renowned for his aesthetic techniques and holistic approach to aging, he is regularly featured in the media as a skin and aging expert. Since releasing his first book, *Turn Back the Clock Without Losing Time*, Dr. Frank has been a clinical investigator, brand ambassador, and consultant for numerous international skincare, technology, and pharmaceutical companies, including the Estée Lauder Companies and Madonna's MDNA SKIN. Recently, Dr. Frank has made significant contributions to the cosmetic dermatology industry with the launch of PFRANKMD—a multi-provider and multidisciplinary bespoke aesthetic healthcare brand. As a board-certified dermatologist, he has lectured around the world and authored several articles for both consumer and medical publications. Dr. Frank is a Clinical Assistant Professor of Dermatology at the Icahn School of Medicine at Mount Sinai Hospital.